Tooth

Decay

How to Heal Cavities and Reverse Tooth Decay

(How I Stopped Tooth Decay and Avoided Dental Surgery With This All Natural)

Claude Hartley

Published By **Phil Dawson**

Claude Hartley

Tooth Decay: How to Heal Cavities and Reverse Tooth Decay (How I Stopped Tooth Decay and Avoided Dental Surgery With This All Natural)

ISBN 978-1-998038-16-9

No part of this guidebook shall be reproduced in any form without permission in writing from the publisher except in the case of brief quotations embodied in critical articles or reviews.

Legal & Disclaimer

The information contained in this book is not designed to replace or take the place of any form of medicine or professional medical advice. The information in this book has been provided for educational & entertainment purposes only.

The information contained in this book has been compiled from sources deemed reliable, and it is accurate to the best of the Author's knowledge; however, the Author cannot guarantee its accuracy and validity and cannot be held liable for any errors or omissions. Changes are periodically made to this book. You must consult your doctor or get professional medical advice before using any of the suggested remedies, techniques, or information in this book.

Table Of Contents

Chapter 1: Tooth Decay

For tooth decay to take location within the first location, there must be the presence of acid around the tooth and food to supply the bacteria. When enamel have no fluoride, the teeth is not able to fight off the buildup of plaque.

When humans have awful hygiene, plaque and tartar are able to buildup on the enamel which makes it much less hard and faster for tooth decay to get up. Bacteria are ever-present within the mouth, however most effective one form of bacteria is responsible for teeth decay and that bacteria may be handed from individual to individual with the aid of kidding or sharing a tumbler.

It can take enamel decay two or three years to do important damage to the teeth. It first is going thru the teeth then to the pulp of the enamel. It has numerous layers of enamel to get via. After it gets via those layers made of dentin, it does not take prolonged for the ones bacteria to break the tooth.

A 2nd type of teeth decay is known as smooth decay and this works with the resource of the bacteria dissolving the tooth and leaving white spots at the tooth. This sort of decay is usually visible in humans below 30 years vintage.

Pit, or fissure, decay is a much more important hassle wherein the decay begins along the grooves of the molars wherein people chew. This micro organism works at a far quicker rate than the others due to the fact that those locations are slim and aren't usually brushed well.

The last type of decay is called root decay and this starts offevolved offevolved offevolved at the floor of the root. This often takes area with middle aged humans fro, dry mouth, increases in sugar levels, and lack of right mouth hygiene. This is the toughest form of decay to prevent and it influences the tooth brief. The teeth needs to be removed upon this diagnosis.

The fine manner to prevent tooth decay is to have it handled in advance than it can unfold, in particular on extra younger enamel. Getting a everyday dentist cleaning is critical. Brush on a each day basis and use mouthwash to kill micro organism. If you take care of your teeth, you may frequently prevent enamel decay from taking area.

When tooth decay takes location, there are various things that take location to the tooth or many problems that can permit micro organism in to motive teeth decay.

Abscesses

Abscesses arise even as the gum line, or moderate tissue across the enamel, fills with a pocket of pus that creates an infection. These are intense situations. When the pulp of a teeth dies from every damage or decay, micro organism broaden and feed at the vain tissue this is left. These micro organism will unfold and form an abscess.

Gum infection moreover can be answerable for forming an abscess. Gum sickness works to cut up the gums from the enamel and go away open gaps. Bacteria can get into the ones gaps and purpose and abscess. These styles of abscesses are going to be greater identifiable as they'll be growing underneath the gums in region of near the jaw line on the basis of the enamel.

Since an abscess is an infection, it's far possible for the contamination to spread to places just like the jaw bone. The micro organism want to make room for the swelling so it could devour into your jaw bone. This will reason the teeth to turn out to be loose and want to be eliminated.

Abscesses are easy to diagnose as they are exceptionally painful, have pretty some swelling inside the gums, and a terrible flavor for your mouth. Your jaw may also moreover harm and you could run a fever as it's far an contamination. These are regularly remoted to the again teeth, however they may be recognized to occur inside the the the front every now and then. The teeth should be extracted to kill the contamination because of the truth the contamination can spread rapid. The dentist can also furthermore perform a root canal to take away lifeless tissues.

Cavities

Cavities are teeth decay and a common problem among humans. Cavities stand up due to the components we eat, hygiene, and fluoride stages in toothpastes. People who have a circle of relatives records of teeth issues may additionally additionally bypass the ones all of the way proper all the way down to their youngsters.

Older adults regularly be troubled with the aid of dry mouth. This places them at higher hazard for growing cavities. Saliva manufacturing kills bacteria, but people growth dry mouth due to infection, remedy, or radiation. People who use tobacco also can enjoy dry mouth because the saliva is being used for the tobacco and not lubricating the mouth.

If cavities aren't handled, they'll be able to wreck the tooth, nerves, create abscesses, and gums. The dentist assessments for cavities at the equal time as you skip for a checkup. With a dental go to, it's miles hard to recognize when you have a cavity.

Food is a big contributor to cavities. Eating lots of sugary components and consuming soda places humans at a better danger for cavities. Foods which is probably excessive in sugar provide meals for the bacteria in plaque. These bacteria will produce acid in order to damage the enamel.

The hollow space takes location while the bacteria get thru the layers of tooth and create a hole within the enamel. If this is going untreated, the idea will become exposed and that is painful. The maximum not unusual locations for cavities to upward thrust up is inside the chewing areas on the again tooth, amongst enamel, or at the gum line as these are the toughest places to brush.

Infections

After a enamel has been eliminated, the micro organism are despite the fact that dwelling inside the mouth, even when you have right hygiene. Infections are common and might take hold after an extraction of a enamel. This is regularly constant through taking antibiotics.

Chapter 2: Gum Disease

Gingivitis is also known as gum illness and is excessive enough to create teeth loss. In adults, gingivitis and periodontal sickness are the most commonplace varieties of gum sickness. The extraordinary manner to fight gum illness is to because it must be brush and eliminate any plaque buildup.

Gingivitis is characterised thru the contamination of the gum tissues from plaque and tartar buildup throughout the gum line. The gums are going to be very sore and can bleed at the same time as brushing. Brushing and flossing must not motive bleeding on a everyday basis. If you have got gum ailment and do not deal with it, it'll bring about periodontal sickness. Periodontal illness is while the bone and surrounding shape of the mouth is destroyed and can't be reversed. This can be very superior gum sickness.

In the begin, you may phrase your gums are pink and sore. It will development slowly and now not produce plenty ache. You may additionally moreover begin to lose teeth and be conscious bleeding to your gums. It is critical to visit the dentist for a regular checkup. A dentist is the handiest person to diagnose this hassle. Depending on how a protracted manner along the illness is, you could now not be capable of opposite the harm.

Wisdom Teeth

These are a third set of molars which can be positioned at the very all over again of the mouth. They do no longer are to be had until approximately 17 to 25 years of age. Many human beings have them removed as they are sitting at angles which can be awful for the mouth or motive ache. If they come in generally, they will be regularly left intact.

Wisdom teeth may be impacted. This manner they may be surrounded with the resource of using strong tissue and cannot come through on their very very own. In those instances, the dentist has to lessen out the tooth as they can't be pulled. To determine the right steps on your expertise teeth, the dentist will take x-rays to gauge the scenario. If they want to pop out, those are executed with the beneficial aid of a dental physician and it could be finished with entire IV anaesthesia or neighborhood numbing. It is typically the choice of the affected individual.

After the extraction, there can be regularly swelling and the dentist will provide pain killers. You will not be capable of consume sure meals and hygiene technique can be stated to nicely deal with the extraction websites.

Dry Sockets

Dry sockets are not life threatening, however they will be quite painful. These regularly arise positioned up-surgical remedy after a teeth has been extracted and occur more on the decrease teeth than higher enamel. Though there may be no way to save you a dry socket, it's going to decrease the hazard if you observe the instructions publish-surgical remedy.

A dry socket occurs on the identical time as a blood clot paperwork and detaches from the wall of the socket. If this clot dissolves, it leaves the bone uncovered to meals and air. The bone itself can end up infected and that may be a very painful state of affairs.

By leaving the dry socket by myself, it'll heal on its non-public after approximately 30 days, but it is going to be a painful time. Antibiotics and prescriptions do now not treatment this trouble both. The dentist can p.C. The socket wherein the dentist packs the socket with medicated gauze. This system is repeated so the socket can heal.

Fractures

When it entails teeth, fractures are the maximum not unusual problem. These cracks appear regardless of the age, however are greater not unusual in humans over 25 years antique. These are painful and may be tough to cope with.

The first kind of fracture is an indirect supragingival fracture. This fracture occurs above the gum line and takes region even as you chunk down on something hard. The fractured a part of the tooth can also moreover break off and the ache is lengthy gone, however if there may be uncovered dentin, it may purpose a few sensitivity pain. The dentist can often restore this with a crown.

The 2nd kind of crack is an indirect subgingival fracture and this takes place an extended way underneath the gum line. Once the fractured piece of teeth breaks off, it commonly remains linked to the gums. The dentist may additionally moreover need to do a root canal to save you future pain and to smooth out the canal. The degree of seriousness for this form of fracture is based upon on how a long way beneath the gum line the fracture goes.

The third kind is the indirect root fracture. This takes region underneath the gums and underneath the bone. If the fracture occurs within the root close to the crown of the teeth, a root canal may be finished to salvage the tooth or the complete teeth want to be eliminated.

The vertical apical root fracture is the last type and they may be difficult to address. This is in which the cease of the inspiration motives extreme ache notwithstanding the truth that the nerve is removed. This is due to direct stress at the jaw bone. A root canal is important to take care of this type of fracture.

Chapter 3: Background On Toothaches

Many humans have felt a toothache earlier than despite the fact that no character has probable ever defined it. It is an intense, painful sensation that originates inside the enamel and spreads into the gums or jawbone. It is often throbbing and traumatic with out a treatment preventing the ache.

This should make exceptionally difficult as it's miles one of the worst pains viable and is normally present. Everything you do is painful from eating to snoozing. Breathing on it, warmth or bloodless food, or truly swallowing reasons immoderate pain. There are outstanding styles of toothaches and masses of exceptional natural treatments which can help to alleviate this ache.

A toothache is described as any ache this is around the tooth, a couple of teeth or the jaw. This may be a sizeable form of ache from severe to most effective a moderate contamination. Just as there are various exceptional forms of toothache, there are numerous one-of-a-kind reasons.

Causes

A toothache may be due to many stuff. The teeth ache is mostly a hallmark of various issues within the mouth. Pain is a manner for the body to sign that some factor is inaccurate. This problem is probably some difficulty as small as allergy, which regularly manifests itself in reactions to temperatures. More than forty million Americans have teeth sensitivity. This is frequently because of a lack of healthy diet regime. If your teeth have turn out to be sensitive to warm and cold beverages, it is a first-rate danger that you are experiencing allergic reaction.

Tooth ache additionally may be a stop end result of teeth whitening. The chemical bleaching is acidic and leaves enamel enamel inclined. This creates an boom in enamel decay and demineralization of the enamel. After whitening, it isn't uncommon for people to experience their tooth are more brittle and touchy. Most over the counter enamel whiteners, regularly those which may be in toothpastes, do not in reality whiten teeth, however worsen the gums as a manner to cause them to greater crimson, giving the advent of whiter of enamel.

There are many styles of toothpaste in the marketplace which may be recommended to deal with tooth allergy. Avoiding irritants like ice cream and heat beverages is also endorsed to stop hypersensitivity.

Hypersensitive toothaches are frequently harassed with a few component referred to as Bruxism. This is because of excess placed on on the tooth from teeth grinding that often takes area at night time. People regularly do not recognize that they'll be doing this of their sleep. Grinding wears down teeth and reasons a separation number of the dentine and pulp of the tooth. Once the dentine receives exposed, the pulp sends a message of ache via the nerve and the mind. This is the equal reason that cavities and cracked enamel are painful while uncovered to air. Allowing microbes to enter the tooth motives sensitivity.

When gum recession takes region, teeth also can turn out to be touchy. This takes vicinity while the protective gum layer that typically covers the dentine recedes away and the a high-quality deal tons much less defensive gum layer is exposed. This method the nerves are toward the ground and react to heat and bloodless temperatures.

Cracked teeth and one-of-a-kind defects in enamel can reason sensitivity, as nicely. Even preservation like fillings or veneers. Eating acidic and candy food can devour away on the fillings of the teeth or enamel. This is corrosion that lets in bacteria into the teeth. This can cause a hollow space or infection within the enamel. This additionally happens is excessive harm is finished to the tooth and the idea is uncovered. When the root gets uncovered to air or meals, the pain may be excessive.

People who've sinus troubles can enjoy ache in their enamel, as well. Excess strain within the head can purpose pain in the tooth. Colds and flu can motive the identical troubles. The ears, nose, and throat are all interconnected so whilst someone is sick, it creates tension in the face and head. A headache or facial tension can create the advent of a toothache. Often times, this may be rectified with a ache comfort like Tylenol or Aspirin.

Gingivitis may be some exceptional purpose for sensitivity. Gingivitis creates a recession within the gum line as tartar builds up across the enamel. This takes place at the same time as human beings do not brush and floss regularly. Signs of gingivitis display up themselves as pink and swollen gums. This infection ends in bleeding of the gums while brushing and flossing. It starts offevolved as regular plague buildup however accumulates over time. This plague develops proper into a yellow-brown colored cement-like substance that accumulates at the bottom of the enamel, near the gum line. This plague buildup is so robust that it calls for a dentist to take away it. It have to be scraped from the tooth.

This is any such trouble due to the fact because the tartar builds up, it's going to push on the gum line, causing it to recede. This manner more of the tooth is exposed and is the precept cause for teeth loss in adults. Poor gum health is the primary purpose for tooth loss in Americans over the age of 35. This is likewise known as periodontal sickness. Of this group, 75 percentage have some form of gum disorder and 60 percentage did no longer apprehend some component approximately proper dental care and 39 percent now not often attending the dentist.

Poor food regimen, excessive sugar content cloth, processed additives, and worrying lifestyles are inflicting extra teeth related problems now than ever in advance than. With a lack of education about the significance approximately dental hygiene, it is no surprise human beings are experiencing intense tooth issues.

The biggest cause for tooth issues is dwelling in our gums. Gums are the most crucial function for healthful enamel. Our gums are chargeable for preserving our tooth of their proper vicinity and anchor the enamel. Once tartar begins to push tooth out in their proper area, micro organism and meals are capable of get into the pockets created via the receding gum lines. This outcomes in deep infections which could cause excessive health troubles for the whole frame.

Gum shrinkage is a large problem. The enamel get evermore uncovered at the same time as this takes place. The teeth receives brittle and motives sensitivity to temperatures. This receives worse as the muse gets inside the path of the surface. Once this occurs, it can not be undone due to this prevention is the first-rate manner to forestall it. The tremendous issue to prevent this form of gum recession is through appropriate brushing. You will need to change your toothbrush every 3 to six months and purchase a medium hardness brush. Many human beings assume they need a tough toothbrush, but this will honestly make the scenario worse and accelerate the shortage of the gums.

As many dentists tell us, ordinary flossing is a requirement. This goes to maintain plague from forming below the gum line. If tartar is going untreated, gum ailment, abscesses, and infections arise. An infection that is going untreated will purpose toxicity inside the blood and require severe scientific hobby.

Attending the dentist often goes to help preserve tartar buildup to a minimal. People get rid of going to the dentist and will anticipate they're tremendous, however someday they have got this terrible toothache that could have been prevented has the dentist visits been more regular. Prevention is the fine answer so it's far vital to no longer do away with going to the dentist. Gum recession does no longer truely take region with age each. There are many technological advances to fight gum loss for a long time.

With the massive technological advancements in dentistry, it is viable to have the smooth gum tissue grafted to the receded areas of the mouth. It is an high-priced business enterprise, however it can help to lessen the effects of the misplaced gums. For a graft to art work, you have to have the right amount of gum tissues nonetheless to be had. Certain sorts of humans are not applicants for this. People who have a hard time recuperation or diabetic might not be the proper candidates for this. Prevention goes to be an awful lot higher than trying to correct the trouble later.

While the consequences of gum recession, tooth loss, gingivitis, and tartar buildup are troubles in and of themselves, the make-up of the buildup at the teeth can tell you loads about your traditional health.

Everything this is going into our mouths makes it into our our our bodies. There is a strong correlation between the calcium buildup on teeth and calcium buildup in arteries. This buildup results in coronary coronary heart illness, strokes, and coronary coronary heart attacks. Angina is an enlarged coronary heart. This can create issues for stiff jaws and toothaches, however it's miles a much large trouble with everyday health. The dentist might also study the tooth, however it could require a go to to a health practitioner for similarly treatment. Sometimes, while humans enjoy a coronary heart attack, they'll experience jaw ache at the left facet.

Another state of affairs that may plague humans is Temporomandibular Joint Disorder, or TMJ. This motives aching within the hinge of the jaw and cheek bones. It can even spread to the ears. This joint is answerable for easy movement of the top and reduce jaws and it can come to be tough to consume, communicate, yawn and is normally gift from tooth grinding.

Not all tooth ache is lousy, it is able to be worrying and every now and then an indication of a few thing extra important that requires clinical attention.

Symptoms

There are many signs and symptoms which you are having a desired toothache from a few issue more important that desires interest. Some of the symptoms can most effective be recognized via a dentist.

The signs and symptoms of big toothache incorporate sharp, taking photographs pains that restrict themselves to at the least one place. This frequently comes and goes and can be sensitivity. It also may be head tension, strain or a teeth being uncovered to air. Other signs of a current day toothache are going to be a throbbing or persistent pain which can linger for a long term.

Chapter 4: Types Of Toothaches

Just as there are distinct reasons for toothaches, there may be one-of-a-type varieties of toothaches, as properly. Each one is a trademark of a selected form of trouble.

A sharp, taking photographs pain may be a hallmark of enamel sensitivity. This can be from placed on and tear or a demineralization of the teeth tooth from brushing. A difficult bristle brush can reason this enamel put on. Gum recession is every other purpose for this sharp, taking snap shots pain. This is due to the fact the inspiration is exposed; it can be painful because of the reality it's far root receives extra air than everyday. A decaying cavity, cracked tooth or abscess can also create this type of ache.

Chronic, lingering pain can be because of nerve damage. Nerve harm can get up from tooth grinding, decay of tooth, or trauma from an harm. Tooth decay can penetrate a teeth and cause intense issues.

Pain when eating is mostly a stop end result of a hollow space, it truly is decaying teeth, or a cracked enamel.

Severe throbbing takes place at the same time as there may be swelling inside the face or lymph nodes. It may be swelling below the jaw due to an abscess. One element is typically tenderer than the opportunity, but jaw ache can be on each elements. This can be a hallmark of infection.

Pain close to the yet again of the jaw wherein the molars are can be many things. It can be an impacted understanding tooth if you have now not had them eliminated. In this situation, the teeth does no longer come through the gum line in part and reasons pain while strain is achieved. It is similar to having little one enamel pushing thru the gums.

Temporomandibular Joint illness (TMJ) or Bruxism is a few other cause this sort of pain can also rise up. Tooth grinding is the purpose for this to rise up and reasons ache because of the extended, long time tension on the jaw bones. It also can have an effect at the facial bones in cheeks or the ear canals.

When you placed your palms in this structure, you may enjoy the relationship a few of the top and decrease jaws. If you place your finger into your ear while chewing, you may sense the motion of the Temporomandibular joint. When there's friction proper here, there may be pain.

No depend what the cause is on your toothache, it is able to be an illustration of a intense health trouble so it's far critical to have any toothache looked at by means of using a dentist.

Natural Cures for Toothaches

There are many natural treatment plans that make it feasible to prevent toothaches without troubles, at domestic. These remedies also can help to reduce any feasible infection in the tooth. Each treatment varies with how lengthy they take to work. Some paintings in a don't forget of mins, others take hours. While those treatments can help to reduce contamination and ache, they do not update the requirement for a dentist.

As a temporary degree for ache comfort, those are a awesome desire. If you still revel in pain, get to a dentist proper away because of the truth it could be a sign of a few detail greater immoderate. There isn't any possibility for dental treatment. Everyone wants to get dental remedy on a everyday basis. To get everlasting remedy, you want to treat the purpose of the pain, not simply the signs and signs and symptoms and signs.

Natural treatments can deal with toothaches with items which you have across the residence. These are clean to put in force at home and provide no difficulty effects due to the fact they're herbal treatments. While those treatments are steady, there are some that pregnant women ought to avoid because of the individual of the substances.

Ice Compress or Mouth Rinse

If your toothache is a stop end result of hypersensitivity, the ones are going to be complicated. Ice works handiest for excessive fine styles of toothaches. If you aren't touchy to cold, ice might also help to alleviate the ache. If the toothache isn't always from sensitivity, it is able to be a signal of contamination and ice may be the extremely good alternative.

Ice is going to artwork at the ache through the use of numbing the affected vicinity and converting the indicators from the nerves which are transmitted to the thoughts. Swelling and contamination are also reduced. This swelling can take vicinity if there's an abscess. There are numerous sports to make the ice art work properly on the ache.

First, start via wrapping an ice cube in a washcloth and run cold water over the fabric for ten seconds. This allows the coldness of the ice dice to come back lower again through the washcloth. Place the cold washcloth on the tooth or close to the teeth.

Another way to make this effective can be to apply an icepack and region it on the affected teeth or outside of the mouth. Put pressure on the region to help get the maximum effect out of the ice.

Within a few minutes, you should sense a remedy within the pain. If you do now not have an icepack, a p.C. Of frozen vegetables will suffice. When you rub an ice cube immediately at the take a look at over the vicinity, it may create at once pain treatment.

If the enamel pain is truely excessive, vicinity the ice dice proper away on your mouth over the affected place. You want to depart it proper proper right here so long as possible. If you may stand it till it's miles completely melted, that is probably outstanding. The longer the ice is there, the extra pain consolation you may get.

Another alternative is to swirl bloodless water on your mouth. This will reduce the pain, but in all likelihood not absolutely do away with it like ice will.

Salt Water Gargle

Salt is one of the oldest remedies for enamel pain. It has been used for added than three,500 years for retaining right and killing bacteria. This is one of the only strategies to treat infection in any wound and perfect for treating teeth pain. Its outstanding bacteria stopping power comes from the capability to attract in bacteria and kill them off.

The method of osmosis includes a lower saline cognizance level moves throughout a membrane of a cell to a higher interest of saline tiers. When the saline moves to a better hobby degree, the bacteria are left in the back of and diet regime off from dehydration. This is why salt is a terrific deliver of preservation and the number one difficulty in mummification of the Egyptians.

The maximum commonplace reason for toothaches is contamination. This can be due to a cracked tooth or missing filling, but decomposed meals takes hold in cracks or infections and micro organism breed.

Chapter 5:Acupressure

This isn't always a recommended treatment for ladies who are pregnant. There are many stress elements all around the body and Ancient Chinese treatments can treat ache thru way of utilizing pressure. This is an possibility remedy that is quite famous. If the pressure factors are focused as it should be, it could provide a fantastic deal of ache remedy for the affected man or woman.

There are many studies which is probably showing that making use of appropriate pressure to high quality points of the body encourages endorphin launch in the mind. Endorphins are the chemicals of the thoughts that decorate painkilling and relieve ache on the internet site.

A unmarried nerve this is located most of the thumb and index finger has the same receptors because the teeth. Applying ice to this specific issue can signal the mind to alleviate ache for the teeth. There are numerous approaches to do this.

The first manner is to place an ice dice in this a part of the hand. To discover the right spot at the hand, search for the fleshy net of the hand that is located at the "L" a part of the hand. It is equidistance among the thumb and index finger. This factor may additionally furthermore reason teeth ache and can also control it. Make fine which you follow ice to this a part of the hand for 10 to 20 minutes. You want to maintain it instantaneous till you enjoy relief.

If the toothache is greater excessive, make an ice bathtub for the hand. This is finished with combining cups of beaten ice with cups of water in a bowl. Put the hand in to the bowl and rub down the strain problem with the opportunity hand for one minute. You do no longer need the hand to get too bloodless. Repeat until the ache within the tooth stops.

Another method is to vicinity strain in this factor of the hand with the other hand. Hold this for 2 to three minutes. This will launch the endorphins to prevent the pain in the tooth. Using the body's very non-public herbal pain relievers may be a eternal manner to save you the ache. Do no longer do that if you are pregnant.

One different place for acupressure is the moderate location throughout the Achilles' tendon on the again of the ankle. Grasp this a part of the ankle for 2 to 3 mins and the pain want to subside.

Garlic Cloves

Garlic is an ancient treatment for many things, predominantly and antiseptic. Ancient cultures like Egyptians, Romans and Greeks used garlic as prolonged within the beyond as three,000 BC. Garlic consists of a compound known as Allicin. Once garlic is overwhelmed, the Allicin is launched and works as an antiseptic and anesthetic. Garlic may be utilized in some of techniques.

The first strategies it to combine one clove of garlic with a sprinkle of salt and create a paste that may be implemented right away to the affected location. Be cautious because of the fact if have a take a look at too much it may create a burning sensation.

The second choice is to weigh down a clove of garlic and blend it with a teaspoon of peanut butter and apply it to the affected vicinity.

The zero.33 preference is to place an entire piece of garlic on your mouth for 1/2-hour. Applying pressure can make this greater effect so pressing at the clove or biting down at the garlic. You need to launch genuinely enough juice that it treats the affected area. You should feel remedy after about 20 mins.

Chewing on garlic can support the immunity common and heal contamination or inflammation in teeth.

Onion

Much like garlic, onion has recovery homes and works as a natural antiseptic. This treatment was used by many early pioneers that came to America and become a remedy for bronchial bronchial asthma and colds. The Chinese believed onions as a way to deal with coughs, congestion, and bacterial infections. The fulfillment of onions as remedies has long beyond so far that the World Health Organization acknowledges onions as a remedy for sure ailments.

To use this remedy, you need to start through setting a piece of onion over the affected enamel that is massive enough to cowl the whole place. Leave this set for half of of-hour to kill micro organism and provide pain comfort. If it's far feasible, lessen off a bit of the onion and bite on it for two or three mins at the affected teeth. This will create antiseptic cleansing of the region and fight pain.

Almond or Vanilla Extract

Both vanilla and almond extract embody alcohol and feature painkilling homes. Vanilla extract does have a higher alcohol content material diploma, however every are effective. This may be executed through using manner of soaking each a cotton ball or a Q-tip soaked inside the extract and done to the affected vicinity or tooth. Within mins, the extract should numb the vicinity.

Oats

Oats are an effective way to draw pus or infection out from an abscess. Take one tablespoon of oats on the affected teeth and chew down gently. Let this set for ten mins and then rinse mouth with a salt water aggregate.

Iodine

Iodine has been used because the early 20th century as a shape of disinfectant for consuming water. When water comes from a inflamed supply, it includes bacteria and iodine is powerful at micro organism elimination. This makes it useful for open wounds, as well. Simply place a drop of iodine of the teeth, but do not swallow it. Leave it for 2 mins after which rinse mouth with water very well.

Hydrogen Peroxide

This desires to be food grade for protection. It works to kill contamination through changing the molecular shape of bacteria. The manner of oxidation destabilizes that molecules of bacteria and that they damage aside so they'll be useless. This is the approach this is motives hydrogen peroxide to foam at the same time as it contacts micro organism. Local pharmacies ought to offer hydrogen peroxide this is food grade.

To use it, swirl round a mouthful of three percent Hydrogen Peroxide then spit it out and rinse severa instances with water to get ache treatment. You also can dilute out the peroxide with the useful aid of combining half of of a pitcher of peroxide to half of a glass of water. Swish it round in the mouth for 30 seconds and spit it out. Then upward push with lukewarm salt water.

Pepper

Almost all kitchens have pepper and it gives ache comfort from toothaches and can lessen the sensitivity teeth can develop. This may be performed by using manner of taking a teaspoon of salt and a punch of pepper. Mix it nicely and vicinity it on the sore teeth. By brushing each day with this type of aggregate can defend teeth in competition to cavities, bleeding gums, awful breath, pain and sensitivity.

Ginger Root

Ginger root is indigenous to India and China and deemed to be one of the worldwide's most vital spices. Ginger is often used for flavor via have healing houses. This aids in digestion, decreasing horrific levels of cholesterol and reduce blood pressure. It is a natural relaxant for arterial walls. As humans age, those partitions constrict and blood go with the float is reduced. Ginger can assist loosen up those arteries to go again regular blood waft.

In both uncooked or powder, ginger root is able to help fight teeth pain. If using powdered ginger, location a teaspoon of powdered ginger and cayenne pepper and upload some drops of water to create a paste. Place this combination on a cotton ball until completely saturated after which practice to the affected teeth. You will want to area the cotton ball absolutely at the enamel as the pepper can worsen the gums. Ginger and Cayenne can art work one after the other, however collectively they may be a awesome possibility.

Raw ginger root can be bought on the grocery keep and may be used to deal with a toothache. Cut the ginger and peel the outer layer of pores and pores and skin then vicinity the ginger at the teeth. If you can chew right all the manner down to keep it in vicinity. This is will lower the ache because the ginger is absorbed into the enamel. If you may chunk the ginger, it's going to desensitize the painful teeth.

Fresh ginger root maintains long time inside the fridge and continues at room temperature as an entire piece.

Vitamin D

Vitamin D deficiencies can cause many issues for human beings at the side of Rickets disorder. A lack of weight loss program D creates weak point in bones, which has a sturdy effect on the health of enamel. Most milk is now fortified with vitamin D. The frame furthermore makes vitamin D at the same time as uncovered to sunlight hours.

Chapter 6: Cloves

Cloves are a treatment that has been implemented for loads centuries as antiseptic and anesthetic. Cloves in each a glowing or dehydrated form with help to prevent toothache pain. The clove may be found decrease returned as a protracted manner as hundred BC in China as a treatment for tooth pain and breathe freshening. The first actual dentists used cloves in oil form to assist combat tooth pain publish extraction. The Eugenol is the element that comes from cloves that is bacterial fighting and a pain killer. Even now, cloves are a exceptional manner to assist manage enamel ache and there are various processes to do this.

The first manner to apply cloves is to apply a glowing or dehydrated clove and located it at the painful teeth or place. Bit down with out problem for about half-hour. If the pain lets you chunk on the clove, gain this. This allows the oils to permeate the teeth and gums. You should have numbness internal only some minutes of chewing

The 2d way to get blessings from cloves is through using clove oil to the spot that hurts with a Q-tip. Avoid using to the tongue or gum region. The clove oil also can have a focused, robust taste this is often unsightly and can get worse soft tissues throughout the enamel. Only leave the oil on for approximately 3 minutes for good enough consequences.

Clove oil have to simplest be used externally and do no longer swallow it. Rinse the mouth with water as quickly as you've got have been given accomplished it and obtained ache treatment. It is not encouraged that people examine greater than applications as clove oil can be poisonous in massive quantities and pregnant girls should not use clove oil.

Tea Tree Oil

Native Aborigine's used tea tree oil as a natural antiseptic within the Australian outback. This occurred prolonged earlier than cutting-edge remedy took keep. Tea tree oil is beneficial because it is able to penetrate deep into the enamel because of this it's miles a brilliant remedy for deep tissues which might be laid low with wounds, contamination and sooths broken tissues while assisting to restore them.

To use tea tree oil to combat contamination and tooth ache, create a mouthwash by using taking three drops of tea tree oil in eight oz... Of water and stir it properly. Swirl a mouthful of the answer for 30 2nd and spit it out. Repeat and rinse your mouth with a lukewarm saltwater answer. Do no longer swallow the tea tree oil. The ache want to be exquisite eased after mouthwashes with the tea tree oil answer. This oil answer can get deep into the gums and numb the nerves which may be sending the pain signals. Tea tree oil is able to kill infections and it could reduce swelling and redness, as properly.

Peppermint

Peppermint is a recognized anti inflammatory that makes use of menthol to heal. As a herbal anesthetic and bactericide, this can be finished to the affected place to offer pain comfort. Menthol is the active element in joint and ache lotions that relieve pain. It is also used to assist humans alleviate their bloodless or flu signs and symptoms and signs and symptoms as a decongestant. From an aromatherapy issue of view, peppermint provides a chilled effect that is soothing. It is a common use for homeopathy.

To use peppermint as a remedy for toothaches, take four grams of peppermint and vicinity them in a coffee mug. Fill it with boiling water and add a teaspoon of salt. Make positive to stir very well and permit it to chill until the mixture is lukewarm. This offers the maximum pleasant houses of the peppermint to be utilized. Swish the solution around on your mouth to get insurance over the area this is affected and swallow. After 10 to fifteen minutes, the ache will depart.

This gets to the supply of the ache and allows relieve pain from inner sources, as well. Just like aspirin, peppermint can artwork from the internal out to treat toothaches, jaw pain, and complications.

Peppermint does not need to be clean for it to art work. It can be dried and actually as powerful. You can percent those leaves round a sore enamel in case you do not want to motive them to proper proper into a peppermint tea. Putting stress at the region through the usage of manner of biting down for 10 to 20 mins is also effective. Chew at the leaves to permit the oils to soak in and then spit them out. This will draw out infections that encompass toothaches and works as a painkiller.

Tea

Tea is one of the maximum ancient remedies for plenty illnesses, which includes toothaches. The Chinese have used tea as a treatment for masses of years. It has often been a treatment for headaches. It also can work as a topical remedy for toothaches. While it is soothing, tea also can offer antibacterial houses by using manner of killing viruses, bacteria, and fungi.

Since tea has many antioxidant homes that come from polyphenols, tea has the ability to fight illness and safety from various ailments like maximum cancers and tumors. To make tea paintings for a toothache, location a normal teabag in a cup of water and microwave for one minute. Remove the teabag even as it's far warm temperature and region it at the affected vicinity. Bite down gently or maintain it in location for 20 mins to get the maximum ache comfort. Green tea works pretty properly, as properly.

Wheatgrass

Wheatgrass is the younger version of without a doubt grown wheat containing chlorophylls. Chlorophylls is a definitely taking vicinity antiseptic and might penetrate deep into the tissues to heal wounds or ulcers which is probably because of infections. Wheatgrass can pull out an contamination via killing bacteria and preventing any inflammation which reduces ache. Wheatgrass is to be had at fitness stores and supermarkets.

Juice from the wheatgrass may be become a mouthwash with only some handfuls of wheatgrass in a juicer. Swirl a mouthful of the wheatgrass juice on your mouth, undiluted, and reputation on the vicinity that is in ache, preserving it to your mouth for 30 seconds earlier than you swallow it.

Wheatgrass has many healing homes even as you drink it as nicely like assisting food plan and stopping teeth decay that might reason the ache within the first area. If the taste is ugly, you may spit it out after rinsing with it. The juice is useful but you could additionally spoil off the shoots of the wheatgrass and chew on them to get the wheatgrass to the website online of the tooth pain.

Cucumber

Cucumber has a immoderate recognition of vitamins C that comes from ascorbic acid makes it an effective anti-inflammatory. It will assist to lessen swelling and draw out bacteria. Cucumbers are smooth to find out and to apply it to a painful enamel is straightforward. Just slice the cucumber in slices which can be half of inch in thickness and chew down lightly on the enamel that is affected. Hold it in area for ten minutes and the ache ought to subside in that quantity of time. If you refrigerate the cucumber, it's going to assist to lessen the swelling as bloodless constricts the blood vessels which motive infection and ache.

Covers

With a tooth that has a massive hollow area, filling, chip, or missing piece, air publicity goes to create critical sensitivity. It might also even growth the possibilities for contamination and pain. When food debris get into the enamel, it is able to with out problems create an infection.

For decreasing pain from an uncovered hole vicinity, chewing a chunk of sugar unfastened gum and urgent it at once to the affected tooth can assist plug the hole space to lessen the air exposure. It is a short seal till you may get to a dentist for a eternal healing. This will maintain meals out of the hollow space and save you infection. It will also lessen the sensitivity to warmness and cold, as nicely.

Including a overwhelmed aspirin to the gum can help reduce the pain. Make high-quality the aspirin does no longer are available in contact with the gums as it is able to purpose burning sensations. Including quantities of garlic, cucumber, onion or sensitive toothpaste can assist to reduce the pain of those teeth illnesses. You do no longer want to bite the gum at the same time as on the enamel.

Asafoetida

Asafoetida comes from a ferula plant that comes as a resinous gum. When the stem of the flowers are lessen, the sap comes out in a resin shape that is frequently used as a flavor for curry based totally definitely totally dishes in Middle Eastern dishes or Indian food. It is often used as a medicinal remedy for masses ailments. It can assist freshen breath, increase digestion and treating teeth pain.

Chapter 7: Dental Corrections For Toothaches

When you have got had been given intense enamel ache, the dentist will decide what is wonderful for the tooth and this may are available a whole lot of treatments.

Root Canals

Root canals are something many human beings already apprehend about and dread. This is a manner wherein the dentist saves the tooth with the useful resource of getting rid of the dry or vain pulp inside the teeth. If it isn't removed, it can cause infection and abscesses. A hole is drilled into the tooth and the nerves are scraped out. This is an extended manner that often has anesthetic associated with it.

Root canals are wanted even as a tooth is considered to be severely decayed. It is a way to address tooth ache and hold the teeth alive. These are extended, high priced strategies, however will save ache within the destiny.

Fillings

Fillings are a common workout for dentistry. This is a way to restore a tooth from a hole area. The dentist receives rid of the decaying vicinity of the enamel and then closes the location to maintain bacteria out and repair the natural shape to the teeth. Fillings can be gold, porcelain, resin or amalgam. There is not one ideal shape of filling.

If the hole space has cracked the tooth or reasons excessive harm, it may require a cap or crown. If the harm gets to the nerve, a root canal is completed. The cap or crown is going on pinnacle of the tooth to keep it collectively and encase the damaged tooth.

Extractions

Extraction includes getting rid of the whole tooth and takes location whilst the pulp of the teeth has died. There are kinds of extraction: clean and complex. Simple extractions contain loosening the gums for the duration of the socket and rotating the enamel thing to element to get rid of it. This is likewise known as pulling a teeth.

A complex extraction consists of a situation wherein the enamel can not truely be pulled out. This involves cutting into the gums and bone to put off a enamel because of the reality it's miles impeded in some manner or the infection has spread too a ways and required in addition elimination.

Many human beings ask approximately pulling their personal tooth. This is never endorsed. It is a painful method that is frequently completed beneath complete anesthesia if no longer numbing. Pulling your very own teeth can result in contamination. The handiest permissible times for pulling enamel are if there is a free child teeth or you be bothered via extreme gum sickness and the enamel is already loose. You have to in no way use implements to drag a enamel. Leave that to the dentist.

Ending Recurring Tooth Pain

When toothaches are regular, it may be quite uncomfortable and interrupt each day existence. There are a few preventative measures that you could take to prevent destiny toothaches.

The first element to do is visit the dentist frequently. The exquisite way to save you a toothache is to make certain that habitual dental care stops toothaches at their sources. The toothache is usually a symptom of some factor else for you to prevent habitual tooth ache, it's far vital to deal with the motive.

The 2d element to forestall ordinary pain is to trade your lifestyle. Lifestyle may be honestly clearly considered one of the largest members to fitness of enamel. The cause for tooth ache is frequently from degradation of the teeth from eating regimen or manner of life. When teeth decline in fitness on a regular foundation, toothaches can be become greater frequent. Many human beings do now not even apprehend a few element is wrong until the toothache appears. This is why tooth decay and gum disorder have been known as silent killers due to the fact they accumulate through the years and feature drastic effects.

Changes to food regimen should make substantial upgrades to the fitness of tooth. By getting extra calcium and phosphate to a food plan can help to defend the enamel of enamel and rebuild the erosion that could have happened. This works via remineralization. The teeth do have the capability to restore themselves.

Many dentists do not allow their sufferers apprehend they could remineralize and restore the tooth of their enamel. Teeth moreover do not need to get weaker as you age. They can get more potent. There are many meals resources to help make tooth stronger because of the truth they may be rich in calcium. Foods like milk, yogurt, cheese, chickpeas, tofu, nuts, oats, cabbage, broccoli, oranges, and turnips.

Most humans want about 1,000 milligrams of calcium in step with day for people who are some time 19 to 50 and getting this advice is as easy as cups of yogurt in keeping with day.

Phosphate is a extremely good story. It takes vicinity in substances like egg yolks, milk, nuts, beans, lentils, wheat germ, soy, oats, and corn. These meals frequently double in phosphate and calcium so thru manner of having one, you have got become the possibility.

Brushing your enamel with baking soda also can assist enhance the fitness of tooth. Avoiding toothpastes that have glycerin goes to help. Baking soda decreases enamel erosion and kills bacteria within the mouth.

Foods with flour and sugar are going to rush up erosion. These ingredients can even boom micro organism that could purpose problems with tooth and gums. By avoiding these ingredients, the tooth are able to rebuild the enamel.

Getting more end end result, veggies, and complete grains to your diet plan get fiber and provide textures that assist smooth the tooth, dispose of bacteria, and smooth off plaque. These foods often have food regimen D which is likewise going to assist teeth from the inner out. Vitamin D comes from fish oil, cheese, and egg yolks. This is in particular essential because of the reality weight loss program D enables to boom calcium absorption.

Brushing and Flossing

Brushing is a few component anyone determined out early on in lifestyles. It is essential to brush nicely and that may be performed in masses much less than mins. Use quick mild strokes, now not difficult pressure while brushing. Spend maximum of some time brushing those hard to collect areas as this is in which plaque will buildup.

You want to trade your toothbrush every six months or extra frequently. As toothbrushes get used, the bristles wear down and are plenty less able to take away plague. Plague paperwork at the gum line and even as it builds up, it effects in gum illness. You will need to brush two times in step with day, particularly after a meal for outstanding effects.

The right toothpaste may additionally make a difference. Get toothpaste that forestalls sensitivity and toothaches. One that stops tartar and gingivitis is great, as properly. The dentist can provide you with an excellent recommendation on toothpaste.

Brushing your tongue at the same time as you brush your enamel goes to promote the destruction of bacteria. The tongue is protected with bacteria and can cause sore throats and Streptococcus. By disposing of the ones micro organism, you're able to stay wholesome.

Just as you need to brush every day, flossing is essential, as properly. You want to do that earlier than bed as that is at the same time as the bacteria that reason plague buildup can rise up for your sleep. Flossing facilitates to save you gingivitis, but you have to floss among teeth and underneath the gum line. This is wherein food and bacteria buildup that motives periodontal disease, abscesses, tooth loss, and gum recession.

At first, flossing can motive tenderness, redness, swelling, and bleeding. As you floss greater frequently, it's going to get plenty less difficult and much much less sensitive. Hard bristle toothbrushes also can do this, however you want to avoid those as they will cause deterioration of the gums.

There are varieties of floss, nylon and single filament. Nylon will come waxed or unwaxed. Nylon floss can shred whereas single filament can't so it is often the better desire for floss so you do no longer get portions caught for your tooth, but both one receives the hobby done.

Sugar loose gum is also going to promote health if you chew it after the last meal of the day. This is going to promote saliva production so micro organism are flushed from the mouth. The body's first line of safety towards micro organism prevention is saliva.

Do no longer devour amongst food because it offers the bacteria a chance to regrow. Bacteria are splendid capable of stay on the food that accumulates at the enamel and gums. Sugary snacks are going to decorate that. You want the enamel to live as clean as feasible in between food and brushings.

By taking those preventative steps, you are capable of decrease the risk of getting recurring toothaches and decorate the enamel, gums, bones, and promote ordinary fitness.

Dental Emergencies

There are many dental troubles that want to be handled proper now. These encompass damaged enamel, teeth out of the socket, knocked out tooth, lip or gum abrasions, and some thing else that offers to be a vital hassle desires to be treated with the resource of a dentist day or night.

Often instances, the teeth may be capable of be located lower back in place so make certain which you have the teeth and it is straightforward. The dentist can will let you understand what option is excellent on your particular dental emergency.

Chapter 8: Preventing And Reversing Cavities With Natural Tooth Care.

Isn't it proper that the handiest manner to restore a hole area is to scrape it out and fill it? Wrong. That's what your dentist tells you, and it is viable that she or he believes it. However, with right vitamins and opportunity care practices, we can heal and red meat up our teeth from the internal out.

Even even though modern tradition has separated dental and clinical practices to the factor wherein coverage coverage is separate, our enamel are however as an entire lot a part of our our bodies as our blood, bones, and organs! Your teeth are located at the prevent of a complicated community of nerves, cells, and tissues that paintings to preserve them healthy.

In fact, the tooth and gums show some of the first symptoms and signs of sickness... You've in all likelihood heard that gum fitness is associated with cardiovascular sickness!

It makes no enjoy to break up your dental health from the rest of your frame's fitness.

We're doing it wrong as a tradition, and it is displaying. According to the National Institute of Dental and Craniofacial Research, there has been an alarming boom in enamel decay for the motive that Nineteen Nineties.

42% of youngsters aged 2 to 11 have dental caries in their primary teeth, and 21% have decay in permanent enamel 40 % of adults aged 35 to forty four have decayed, missing, or filled enamel MOST SHOCKING: There is simplest a 1% lower in decayed, lacking, or filled enamel at the same time as the demographic falls underneath the poverty line

The United States spends extra than $20 billion in line with 12 months on dental care.

Why isn't always the fee of cavitation decreasing as generation advances, get admission to to dental care increases, and knowledge about teeth fitness turns into greater appreciably to be had?

Surprisingly, the solution may be right in the front people: weight-reduction plan. It can not be a twist of fate that the upward thrust in cavities coincides with the upward thrust in processed food intake in our speedy-food lifestyle.

If you eat a healthy diet plan and also have new cavities every time you visit the dentist, it is probably no longer because of horrible dental hygiene. Almost half of of of all American adults have cavities in their teeth.

The percent of kid's teeth with cavities is increasing at an alarming charge, which defies exact judgment if it's miles clearly a don't forget of brushing and flossing. Dr. William Bowen, D.D.S., Ph.D., Professor of Dentistry at the University of Rochester, is a international expert on enamel decay. In a bit of writing posted in 2000, he expresses his difficulty approximately the upward push in tooth decay.

"Adults have ninety five% of the time cavities. Some people take into account that the trouble has been solved, however this is absurd. There is not any outstanding disorder I apprehend of in which it is taken into consideration achievement while 50 percent or smore of the populace although has the illness."

Dental caries in youngsters had been step by step declining at some level within the Seventies and Eighties, however new research shows that cavities have risen dramatically in modern-day years, growing from a mean of two cavities in ten-12 months-old's' mouths to a few!

That's a 33% increase! All these cavities cannot be attributed to horrible dental hygiene. When your nicely brushed tooth show symptoms of dental caries, it's far maximum likely because your teeth aren't getting the vitamins, they require to remineralizer and live robust.

Chapter 9: What Are Cavities Exactly, And How Do We Get Them?

A cavity is a hole within the enamel of the tooth. Cavities are also known as "dental caries." Bacteria get into the hollow inside the tooth and rot out the teeth pulp, eventually killing the tooth. Okay, it truly is straightforward, but the larger query is: what motives cavities? Herein lies the problem.

Modern dentistry adheres to the medical precept that cavities are typically due to bacteria on the teeth. The reality is this idea turned into observed through the use of popular vote a long time within the beyond and has but to be definitively tested. Meanwhile, exceptional properly-supported theories, along with the concept that enamel decay is prompted by and large with the beneficial aid of negative diet in location of acid or micro organism, had been debunked.

Dr. Weston Price, a trailblazing dentist, superior his vitamins principle after reading cultures with each low or immoderate expenses of dental caries. He focused an entire lot of his studies on primitive people who've been now not exposed to the posh of consolation meals, as those human beings appeared to have the extremely good enamel and regular fitness. He placed something awesome via manner of paying near interest to their diet and dental hygiene: individuals who ate a traditional food regimen excessive in fats-soluble vitamins and minerals with very little processed grains and sugars had nearly no cavities.

Wait, there may be greater: people who ate this manner had wholesome, strong tooth regardless of their dental hygiene! Even if their dental hygiene have come to be actual, cultures which have been brought to modern comfort meals which consist of jams and jellies, pastries, white bread, and ample sugary end result had an prolonged way worse tooth! Dr.

Price went at once to the lab to test his speculation that terrible vitamins caused cavities, attempting out substances for dietary content material and attractive in a sequence of research to expose his concept.

Price studied a hard and fast of horrible children who lived in maximum cases on "exceedingly sweetened strong espresso and white bread, vegetable fats, pancakes manufactured from white flour and eaten with syrup, and doughnuts fried in vegetable fat" in a unmarried case.

This diet plan lacked the fat-soluble vitamins and minerals required for robust tooth... And those youngsters had decayed enamel to reveal for it!

Dr. Price have been given right down to remineralizer the children's teeth, heal cavities, and save you destiny dental caries with the resource of nourishing their our bodies. This may feature a robust foundation for his hypothesis. These malnourished children were fed a nutrient-wealthy eating regimen for one meal six days each week for 5 months for the purposes of the have a take a look at.

Dr. Price describes the hole area-reversing menu in this excerpt from his groundbreaking ebook, Nutrition and Physical Degeneration: A Comparison of Primitive and Modern Diets and Their Effects:

The following food were included within the vitamins supplied to these kids in this single meal. At the start of the meal, 4 ounces. Of tomato juice or orange juice and a teaspoonful of a combination of equal elements of a totally immoderate vitamins herbal cod liver oil and an especially excessive nutrients butter had been given. They had been then given a bowl containing approximately a pint of a completely rich vegetable and meat stew, made in huge

73

detail from bone marrow and fine cuts of clean meat: the pork changed into commonly broiled one after the other to preserve its juice earlier than being chopped very outstanding and brought to the bone marrow meat soup, which constantly contained finely chopped greens and lots of very yellow carrots; For the following route, they served cooked fruit with very little sugar and rolls made from freshly floor complete wheat and unfold with excessive-weight loss plan butter. Every day, the wheat for the rolls grow to be ground glowing in a motorized espresso mill. In addition, each toddler obtained glasses of easy complete milk. The menu have end up modified from daily with the resource of manner of substituting meat stew, fish chowder, or animal organs.

The children's dental caries miraculously stopped, and x-rays located that their tooth had been restoration and strengthening! Dr. Price maintained his speculation through this and particular research that no longer exceptional is enamel decay due to malnutrition, but that it is able to furthermore be averted and reversed thru right nutrients.

In the give up, filling cavities does not heal enamel. Nourishing substances assist teeth heal. Fillings, in truth, hinder the proper go together with the flow of nutrients to the teeth. A filling will cast off and stop the decay, however it's going to ultimately kill the tooth. When you visit the dentist and discover that you want an vintage filling changed, you'll see evidence to that impact... Worse but, many root canals are completed on formerly crammed teeth! While fillings may be useful in intense instances of degradation, they may be most effective a short repair for a deeper-seated trouble. To make smooth, I am no longer claiming that proper nutrients will cause new enamel material to develop to fill in gaps due to dental caries.

Just like your bones, as soon as a teeth fragment is misplaced, it is prolonged long past.

When your frame is well nourished with fats-soluble vitamins, your enamel will harden and flip glassy in the course of the cavities, shielding the pulp interior from bacteria and infection. This efficaciously seals your tooth, and your teeth is probably sturdy enough to resist future caries.

Chapter 10: The Essential Diet For Tooth Health.

I can let you know all I need that the right diet plan can heal your enamel, but what precisely is the right diet? We are inundated with diet plans ranging from low-fats and vegan to high-protein and coffee-carb. We have food plan books with thin celebrities on the cover and others with six-% abs. The term "wholesome food regimen" can be enormously confusing.

For the features of this ebook, we are able to limit our talk to a healthy eating plan that promotes wholesome tooth. However, because of the fact your whole frame is satiated with nourishing vitamins and minerals from:

•sparkling and cooked greens, your tooth fitness improves on this plan.

•Meat from pasture (collectively with organ meat), fowl, and eggs

•pastured-raised raw and fermented dairy bone broth

•seafood and cod liver oil

•Healthy tooth, healthful frame.

This is a holistic method that has been used for masses of years in japanese and traditional medical exercise but has been misplaced to trendy civilization. How does it function? The mechanism for enamel healing thru vitamins is easy.

Your teeth are made from 4 important additives: enamel, dentin, pulp, and cementum.

Enamel: This is the difficult layer on the outdoor of the teeth's crown. It is the body's toughest substance, and it is required to address all the chewing we do every day. Modern dentistry believes that teeth teeth isn't always able to withstand acid, which eats holes via it if left unchecked.

Dentin: This layer is like bone and is positioned just under the teeth. Because of its softer composition, it may distribute the strain of every bite.

The pulp is the enamel's innermost layer. It is the smooth substance that homes the nerves and feeds the relaxation of the enamel. When a teeth decays, the pulp starts offevolved offevolved to rot away.

Cementum: This is the cloth that surrounds the enamel's root and connects it to the bone. When the body is satiated with the right variety of fat-soluble nutrients and minerals, it's going to send the vitamins to the pulp of the teeth, to be able to then supply the tooth, dentin, and cementum with what they require to reinforce and heal. This is known as remineralization.

However, if the body is depleted of these important vitamins or is not capable of soak up them, the enamel are the final to build up them.

According to Dr. Price's observations, the cultures with the worst instances of cavitation ate a food plan low in fats-soluble nutrients A and D in addition to essential tooth-constructing minerals.

Meat fed on green grasses, further to free-range chook and duck eggs, raw milk, soups crafted from boiling marrow bones, and sparkling seafood, provide the frame with precise enough portions of these fats-soluble vitamins and minerals (together with phosphorus), which stimulate the glands and supply vital nutrients to the teeth. The Big Food Industry's bottom line and our fairly sensitive taste buds now dictate what we eat. We have come to be highly awful in our our bodies, minds, and mouths as our manner of life shifts a ways from herbal, entire foods and closer to a food regimen in big part made from chemical substances and processed food-merchandise.

ORGAN MEATS:

Perhaps you or your parents grew up ingesting liver and onions. Most of us now turn up our noses on the concept of ingesting an animal's inner organs. The livers, hearts, brains, intestinal walls, blood, and pancreas of humanely raised free-variety animals, however, are full of crucial vitamins for not handiest tooth health, however whole-body properly-being.

Organic liver consists of greater than 4 hundred% of the USDA's endorsed each day allowance of fats-soluble Vitamin A and 30% of the endorsed every day allowance of Vitamin D, similarly to a healthy dose of phosphorus and notable minerals. These nutrients are essential inside the technique of tooth remineralization.

Primitive cultures, together with Native Americans, diagnosed the significance of eating the whole animal. They could roast and eat every organ, in addition to crack the bones for the nutrient-dense marrow. In truth, kids had been regularly fed marrow broth as a complement to or substitute for their mom's milk.

If you're apprehensive approximately cooking liver, try this clean trick: Make a meatloaf with grass-fed floor pork, onion, a free-range egg, and some ounces. Of finely chopped liver. Cook as general, or shape into patties and cook dinner dinner as you will a burger or meatballs.

The meat mixture's mixed textures will mask the smoother texture of the liver, and the flavors will mixture nicely. You can frequently boom the amount of organ meat for your mixture as you get used to the strong, earthy liver flavor.

BONE BROTH:

Contrary to famous belief, bone broth is not as gross as it appears. It's definitely a broth made thru the use of slow-cooking unfastened-range, grass-fed animal bones, or whole fish or crustacean carcasses.

Bone broths are immoderate in minerals like calcium, phosphorus, magnesium, sulfur, fluoride, sodium, and potassium. These minerals, especially phosphorous, are required for the rebuilding of the mineral shape of the teeth.

I advise ingesting or consuming 2 - 3 cups of bone broth in keeping with day to attack cavities from the inner out. It may be used to make a hearty stew or in reality sipped from a mug. In any case, gelatin, fats-soluble vitamins, and minerals are entering your body to aid in the rebuilding gadget.

Simply vicinity the bones or entire carcass of a loose-variety fowl, bovine marrowbone, or fish carcass into the gradual cooker with a sprint of vinegar to make bone broth. Fill halfway with easy water and sea salt (non-compulsory). Set the sluggish cooker to low, cover, and go away to cook dinner dinner for twenty-four to 48 hours.

When refrigerated, real bone broth turns into gelatinous and makes superb thick soups and gravies, similarly to bases for traditional soups like fowl and vegetable or beef-mushroom. Remember to keep away from the usage of noodles or distinct grains for your soups, however diced vegetables are nice!

COD LIVER OIL:

Fermented cod liver oil is type of a liquid dentist, however an entire lot much less terrifying. (Who does no longer cringe a touch on the equal time as the dentist pulls out that scraper?) With specifically centered fat-soluble vitamins A & D, simply 12 teaspoon 2 - three instances a day can relieve enamel pain proper now. Why?

Because you are sending a flood of vitamins on your teeth, which might be crucial for structural repair.

STOP: Don't rush out for your neighborhood fitness meals shop or Amazon to shop for a bottle of cod liver oil virtually however. It is important to bear in mind that not all cod liver oil is the same. Fermented cod liver oil isn't subjected to the high temperatures commonly used within the processing of commercial oils.

Heat processing destroys truly taking location eating regimen D, which should then get replaced with synthetic weight-reduction plan D, which is essentially insoluble within the human frame.

Green Pasture's Blue Ice Fermented Cod Liver Oil, available on-line on the codliveroilshop.Com, is one of the maximum reliable belongings of fermented cod liver oil. The net web website online suggests combining cod liver oil with immoderate nutrition butter oil... Which leads us to the subsequent food in your enamel-health diet regime.

BUTTER OR GHEE FROM GRASS:

Remember whilst butter come to be the awful guy? Well, delicious, creamy, fatty butter isn't virtually harmless. Those hunks of diminished butter located in most grocery store refrigerators will NOT assist heal your tooth.

Factory-farmed dairy cannot even feed a calf, no longer to mention a human.

Commercial butter is crafted from milk pumped from grain-fed, constrained cows which might be commonly given hormones and antibiotics. It lacks what Dr. Price referred to as Activator X, a assets positioned excellent in dairy from cows grazed on hastily growing grasses within the spring and early summer season. This grass-fed butter is a wealthy yellow in color and excessive in fat-soluble nutrients A, K, and E.

It has an super ratio of Omega-6 to Omega-three fatty acids, and it includes the enigmatic "Activator X." "Many youngsters have teeth decay even even as the use of entire milk," in step with Dr. Price's research, "in element due to the fact the milk is just too low in vitamins content material fabric, because of the inadequacy of the meals given to the cows."

He additionally says that grass-fed butter is "usually numerous times as immoderate in fats-soluble activators, together with vitamins A and D, as butter constituted of stall fed farm animals or farm animals on poorer pasture." He determined that folks that ate a weight loss program wealthy in grass-fed butter had nearly no cavities, and that the rate of dental caries decreases within the course of the spring and summer season on the equal time as butter is crafted from the milk of cows grazing on extra youthful inexperienced grasses.

This is because of the reality the deep yellow pastured dairy consists of "Activator X," a issue that turns on the frame's ability to absorb minerals.

Mineral absorption improves teeth mineralization.

If you're lactose illiberal, you could replacement ghee for the butter.

Ghee is clearly clarified butter that has been heated and skimmed of the water and milk solids. It is lactose and casein loose, and it offers a scrumptious taste for your elements. Furthermore, it improves nutrients absorption. Remember to use natural and grass-fed ghee, which may be positioned at maximum health meals shops.

Alternatively, you could make your personal ghee from pastured butter: In a Dutch oven or certainly one of a kind oven-steady dish, region a pound of natural, pastured butter (which incorporates Kerrigold). Preheat the oven to 250°F and bake for about an hour.

Check the ghee at this point; it ought to be very bubbly and browning on the bottom. Continue baking for every different half of of-hour, or until the lowest is slightly toasted however no longer burned.

Remove the ghee from the oven and set aside to sit back barely so it can be dealt with. Set a exquisite mesh sieve over a big bowl and line it with a couple layers of cheesecloth or a smooth muslin fabric. Pour the ghee via the cheesecloth, gathering the solids within the cloth as you go. Fill a smooth Mason jar halfway with smooth liquid ghee and hold in a fab, dry place.

If neither of those alternatives attraction to you, you can always complement your each day weight-reduction plan consumption with Green Pasture's excessive nutrition butter oil.

FERMENTED FOODS:

Eating raw veggies is not better for you. Just because you could eat raw broccoli does no longer suggest you are more healthful; it in reality technique you can chew very well.

Sauerkraut can be utilized in location of the raw broccoli slaw, that's tough to digest. Fermented ingredients, along with raw milk kefir and yogurt, sauerkraut, kimchi, pickles, and kombucha, contain enzymes that start the approach of breaking down food before it even reaches your mouth. This is extensive due to the fact fermentation allows nutrient absorption inside the body.

Probiotics are active cultures found in actual, historically fermented ingredients that sell the growth of healthy bacteria in the gut and due to this increase the absorption of essential vitamins which consist of B vitamins, which we already understand are essential for teeth remineralization.

Chapter 11: Getting Rid Of Grains And Sugar.

How many parents declare that their youngsters simplest devour white food? Pasta, bread, pastries, potatoes, sugar... All nutritionally devoid food that do more to harm your fitness than nourish it. But I can permit you to understand proper now that casting off them out of your existence is much less tough than you believe you studied whilst you understand the harm they are inflicting.

Your dentist is in component correct. Avoiding sugary snacks and grain merchandise is sound advice, but possibly no longer for the motives your dentist shows.

THE WHOLE GRAIN FALLACY: In the early 1900s, the American Dental Association proposed that acids for your teeth had been the premise cause of gum sickness. While this principle have become primarily based completely totally on clinical research, it have become no longer genuinely tested and want to no longer have trumped distinctive theories on the time. The Acid Theory, on the other hand, emerge as familiar as truth and has due to the reality ruled dental practices inside the evolved worldwide.

Drs. Edward and May Mellanby, a husband-and-partner crew, have been reading the results of complete grains on dental caries and the development of rickets across the equal time that Dr. Price emerge as learning the relationship among vitamins and rot in the early 1900s.

We are introduced about consider that whole grains are beneficial to our fitness. Paleo dieters keep away from all grains for lots of motives, the primary health gain being a reduction in low-grade inflammation.

A secondary, however no much less crucial benefit of getting rid of grains from the weight loss plan is improved absorption of fats-soluble vitamins, which are essential for protective and recuperation tooth.

The Mellanbys determined that unsoaked entire grains are immoderate in zhytic acid, which efficiently inhibits the absorption of critical vitamins and minerals along with weight-reduction plan D, calcium, and phosphorus at some point of their huge research at the reason and remedy for rickets.

Remember, these are the rules of wholesome enamel remineralization. Rickets is also due to a scarcity of those vitamins and minerals, and it regularly consequences in skeletal deformation, bone fractures, muscle weak spot, and dental troubles.

Rickets have become a plague among impoverished kids at some degree inside the early twentieth century famine. Even our wealthy children for the time being are nutritionally terrible. The handiest difference is that their malnutrition has manifested in their mouths in desire to the general kind of rickets symptoms and signs and symptoms and signs and symptoms.

By putting off grains from the diet plan, you increase absorption of fat-soluble vitamins and minerals, resulting in stronger, greater healthy enamel that could resist acids and the micro organism that results indefinitely.'

THE HARD TRUTH ABOUT SUGAR

We are all aware that sugar is horrible for us. It makes us fat, ill, light, depressed, and moody, and it motives teeth decay. So why are we able to devour it in such absurd portions?

Americans ate up over ten million metric lots of sugar in 2013. To located it each exceptional way, it's far among 80 and one hundred pounds of sugar constant with individual consistent with yr. Can you don't forget eating almost half of a pound of sugar each few days?

If you're like the common American surviving on the cutting-edge-day weight loss plan, you are doing exactly that. No, you are not hiding below the table with a bag of sugar and a huge spoon.

Sugar is hidden in all the processed consolation elements which have modified the sluggish-cooked real meals that were the diet plan mainstay of preceding generations.

White sugar has been stripped of any nutrients it is able to have as quickly as contained earlier than being focused until it is extraordinarily candy. While soda, cookies, sweet, and ice cream account for half of your not unusual sugar consumption, the relaxation is hidden in ingredients you can in no manner suspect—yes, even "natural" and "natural" additives. Sugar is added to pretty a few components, which encompass pasta sauce, fish sticks, catsup, soy and almond milks, soups, breads, cereals, and masses of others.

Our modern-day processed food regimen is loaded with it; delivered processed sugars can be found in 34 of the 600,000 grocery devices inside the commonplace grocery keep!

But you look at the label, and there may be no factor out of "sugar!" Right. That's how sugar hides right inside the the front of your eyes. Sugar has as much as fifty-six aliases. Among the alternative names for sugar are:

brown rice syrup • excessive fructose corn syrup • fructose • lactose • maltodextrin • malt syrup • dextrose • demarara sugar • molasses • raw sugar • sorbitol • treacle

Just as it'd now not say "sugar" on the label does not propose it's far sugar-loose.

That is the difficult element. Even concentrated grape or apple juice has the identical impact in your frame as natural sugar.... So positioned down the ones all-natural gummy fruit snacks and update them with a pint of strawberries!

Why is sugar so terrible for you? Traditional dentistry, as a substitute, will depend upon the acid and bacteria concept. You've likely been recommended through the usage of your dentist no longer to suck on tough candies or drink soda because of the fact the sugar will sit down down in your teeth and chew a hollow thru your teeth, allowing bacteria to infect the enamel pulp and rot your tooth. Does this sound familiar?

This is accurate, but it is also deceptive. A simply healthy and nourished teeth can withstand the sugar invasion indefinitely. Dr. Miller, the medical doctor who evolved the acid concept of cavitation, said that a wonderfully wholesome enamel ought to withstand cavitation indefinitely. The trouble is that sugar does now not sincerely sit down down down for your tooth. It additionally enters your frame. When you combine the sugar to your mouth with the sugar absorbing into your frame, you get a monster.

Unlike sugar's more healthy counterpart, glucose, that is transformed into power inside the frame, sugar and all of its pseudonyms are in the long run processed inside the liver. If you eat the commonplace of 80-one hundred kilos of processed sugar in step with 12 months, you will be very ill.

•If your liver isn't always breaking down the ones vitamins, they may not achieve your enamel.

•If the vitamins do now not attain your tooth, they'll become malnourished and inclined.

•When your enamel are malnourished and inclined, they can not face up to the sugars which might be sitting on them.

•As a stop end result, a vicious cycle of sugar-malabsorption-hollow space repeats itself.

The food enterprise, which is sort of clearly advocated with the aid of income, is aware what it's miles doing by way of stuffing products with sugar—it's miles developing addictions.

The more sugar you devour, the more you choice, and in the long run, the greater in their product you could buy. We have allowed a clean deliver-and-call for cycle to essentially change the manner we eat and feed our families.

We have grown familiar with greater sweetness in our meals than nature supposed. Our taste buds are the use of our options, that is a lousy hassle. An overburdened liver no longer most effective contributes to enamel decay, however it moreover converts sugar right now into fats in choice to converting it into usable energy.

So, the easy equation is as follows: sugar causes micro organism to offer teeth-ingesting acid PLUS sugar prevents the absorption of demineralizing vitamins = fragile, malnourished tooth which is probably susceptible to decay.

When your dentist advises you to keep away from sugar, you will recognize why—now not surely one stop of the cycle. Consider it... If sugar is excellent accountable for bacteria ingesting holes to your tooth, you need to be splendid brushing it off... However, the skyrocketing boom in the fee of dental caries in cultures that consume a present day, processed diet plan demonstrates that it genuinely does now not paintings that manner.

Chapter 12: Teeth Health Homeopathy.

The word "homeopathy" comes from the Greek terms for "like" and "struggling." Homeopathic practitioners declare that homeopathy dates to four hundred B.C., whilst Hypocrates prescribed very small doses of mandrake root to remedy mania, notwithstanding the truth that big doses of mandrake root motive mania.

Doesn't that sound ridiculous? If you consider this, you are not by myself.

Since its inception, homeopathy has been scrutinized. It's been labeled as quackery, and it isn't whatever more than a placebo effect. Thousands of human beings across many cultures, but, swear with the aid of manner of it and use it on a everyday basis to heal their our bodies, minds, and tooth.

What exactly is homeopathy? As within the case of mandrake, very diluted quantities of a substance are given to heal precisely what a bigger dose might also moreover exacerbate. Homeopathic treatments are created with the aid of diluting a substance in alcohol or distilled water until only some or no molecules of the right substance stay. This diluted solution is then administered to heal a selected sickness, usually in pill shape this is held underneath the tongue.

Samuel Hahnemann revived this loads-yr-vintage exercise inside the early 1800s.

11 He proposed his idea of "like remedies like" after looking at that a medication designed to treatment a illness in an inflamed character frequently reasons comparable signs and symptoms and signs and signs in a healthful individual.

When Hahnemann have turn out to be developing his homeopathic mind and formulating treatments, well-known scientific workout blanketed an prolonged list of dangerous capsules and chemical compounds, collectively with opium and viper's blood. Bloodletting and purging were moreover commonplace.

Hahnemann believed that those sincerely barbaric but broadly practiced scientific practices were dangerous in place of restoration—in fact, many human beings died because of painful medical treatment at the time. This is most likely why a few people began to reveal to Hahnemann's homeopathic techniques, which centered on low doses of unmarried "medicinal drugs" or remedies as an possibility to the almost barbaric practices that often prompted signs worsening or maybe demise.

Hahnemann believed that sicknesses had a nontangible, spiritual outstanding that his homeopathic remedies can also want to address.

The perception that the lower the dosage of a treatment, the greater effective it is, is the second one precept that distinguishes homeopathic method from current-day-day clinical exercise. Therefore, the actual substance is so diluted that it's far often handiest the "essence" of that substance that remains inside the solution.

Homeopathy has spread during the area as an opportunity to mainstream remedy because Hahnemann posted his ebook of sixty 5 homeopathic treatments, Materia Medica Pura, in 1810. Despite the dearth of medical proof to aid the efficacy of homeopathy, tens of hundreds of thousands of people flip to this gentler healing approach: "According to the 2007 National Health Interview Survey, which covered an intensive survey of Americans' use of complementary fitness practices, an expected three.Nine million adults and 910,000 children used homeopathy within the previous three hundred and sixty five days." These figures consist of the usage of "homeopathic" over the counter products in addition to visits to a homeopathic practitioner. Adults paid $2.Nine billion out of pocket for homeopathic capsules and $100 and seventy million for visits to homeopathic practitioners."

Homeopathy's holistic view of the body is regular with our plan to address our teeth as an crucial part of our commonplace being, in desire to as a separate entity requiring a very special clinical practice and method.

Chapter 13: Getting Rid Of Toxic Toothpaste.

When you stroll into the grocery shop and test the toothpaste aisle, you will be aware hundreds of claims that this one will whiten your tooth or that one will reinforce your teeth. What none of that smart packaging famous is the laundry list of toxic chemical materials that fill the tube. Even if you're brushing, rinsing, and spitting out the toothpaste, those pollution are absorbed thru your gums nearly right away.

The following are a number of the toxic chemicals determined in plenty of commercial toothpastes. Are you greatly surprised? If you've got ever have a look at a toothpaste label, you may study that it in reality states: DO NOT SWALLOW. This is because of the truth swallowing this product—which, preserve in mind, is supposed to be positioned in the mouth—may be volatile.

Diethanolamine (DEA) is a foaming agent found in masses of private care products, consisting of shampoo, hand cleansing cleaning soap, shave cream, and (superb, toothpaste). Apparently, we love foamy matters. While the bubbles may make you revel in such as you are becoming a higher easy, the chemical DEA is surprisingly unstable on your fitness and undermines the purpose of the use of toothpaste inside the first area—in the long run, it is not correct for tooth health! Why? Because DEA interferes with everyday kidney and liver characteristic.

As previously mentioned, right kidney characteristic is important for processing the minerals required to deliver nutrients to the teeth. If kidney function is impaired, tooth will no longer remineralizer properly.

Triclosan is an antibacterial agent commonly observed in toothpaste. While its toxicity isn't always specially aimed at disrupting features associated with tooth fitness, we now apprehend that healthful teeth are most effective one a part of a wholesome frame. Teeth are often the number one to show signs and symptoms of disease at the same time as the relaxation of the immune device is attacked or suppressed.

Triclosan is a pesticide, and constant with the united states Environmental Protection Agency (EPA), ingestion or exposure to this volatile chemical is risky to human fitness. Furthermore, triclosan is a member of the chorophenol class of chemical substances, which may be suspected of inflicting most cancers.

These days, sodium lauryl sulfate and sodium laureth sulfate seem like in nearly the whole thing you scrub, rub, or squeeze onto or into your frame. The Environmental Working Group's (EWG) Skin Deep splendor database lists severa excessive and mild worries with the ones sulfates, which encompass contamination with 1,4 Dioxane (a identified carcinogen) at some point of the manufacturing way, pores and pores and pores and skin, eye, and lung contamination, and organ tool toxicity. When reading labels, be careful because of the truth this toxin is probably hiding inside the returned of a apparently harmless call: sodium salt.

Propylene Glycol is a common surfactant in toothpaste... And it is also in antifreeze! Propylene glycol isn't pleasant a pores and pores and skin irritant, however it is also a ability neurotoxin with the capacity to harm purpose organs, regular with its Material Safety Data Sheet.

When you begin your day with a mouthful of enterprise toothpaste (even though it claims to be more "natural" and costs two times as loads), you have come to be geared up your frame for a breakdown in advance than you've got even had breakfast! However, we had been socialized to trust that the ones products are an critical a part of our oral hygiene regular.

While it's far proper that you must preserve your enamel and mouth easy, I can guarantee you that there are higher options.

TEETH BRUSHING WITH CLAY

I'm not suggesting you're taking a clump of your children' modeling clay and start scrubbing your enamel with it. That will be disgusting and useless.

When discussing teeth care, the form of clay we are regarding is Calcium Bentonite Clay Powder—a food-grade clay that can be bought at most health food shops or, of direction, ordered on-line.

The fitness blessings of calcium bentonite clay had been stated and used by many cultures for hundreds of years, most effective to be replaced with the resource of the use of artificial chemical substances in our most present day civilized statistics.

Because clay is essentially a mixture of minerals, metal oxides, and herbal rely, it has severa fitness benefits now not best for the tooth but additionally for the digestive tool. Calcium bentonite clay has the subsequent dental health benefits:

•Toxin absorption and elimination

•Remineralization of the tooth

•Tooth sharpening skills.

Clay toothpaste is not possibly to be determined along Colgate at your nearby grocery keep. However, Earthworks makes a excellent clay toothpaste that may be bought at maximum health meals shops or ordered on line. It carries resultseasily identifiable factors along side clay and crucial oils, and it employs xylitol to mask the muddy taste of raw clay powder. Xylitol is generally observed in sugar-loose gums and baked gadgets, and it has lately been lauded via mainstream dentistry as a strong tool within the fight in opposition to enamel decay. The notable xylitol is made from birch bark, but maximum business grade xylitol is made from corn cob.

Check the label and inquire approximately the supply of the xylitol, as disposing of corn from the diet is critical for every body, but in particular for those who've unique corn allergies.

Making your very non-public clay toothpaste is simply quite easy and less expensive even as in evaluation to shopping for it ready-made... As is the case with the majority of Homemade ingredients and frame care products. To get you began, here's a easy recipe:

RECIPE FOR CLAY TOOTHPASTE

This herbal toothpaste need to be stored in a pitcher box with a respectable-fitting lid.

Avoid the usage of plastic baggage or containers because of the reality the clay may be very absorbent and can absorb toxins from the plastics.

Ingredients:

•four tbsp. Calcium Bentonite Clay Powder

•four teaspoons filtered water

•2–four drops mint extract (or one-of-a-kind critical oil) (non-obligatory)

•2 – 4 tbsp birch xylitol, to taste

Gently integrate all factors until a easy paste bureaucracy, adjusting water and clay as had to gain the preferred consistency. This recipe can without problems be doubled or tripled. Start with a small kind of vital oils and xylitol and taste as you pass. You can usually add more if vital!

*If you do no longer need to apply xylitol or do now not have get admission to to it, sweeten the paste with a small quantity of natural liquid stevia or crushed dried stevia leaf.

Scoop a small amount of clay toothpaste onto the give up of your moist toothbrush to apply. Brush your tooth with the paste in a mild round motion, paying unique hobby to areas of state of affairs and along the gum line.

Spit and graceful with filtered water. This is an elective step due to the reality all the materials are healthful for human consumption and useful on your digestive and immune structures.

TOOTH SOAP BRUSHLING

You possibly partner "cleaning cleaning soap in the mouth" with a punishment for saying some component beside the point.... It emerge as not a pleasing enjoy. However, making your very personal teeth cleaning soap isn't always most effective a enjoyable experience; it is able to moreover help hold your enamel strong and wholesome.

From Birth to Death: Good Teeth Dr. Gerald Judd, PhD suggests using bar cleansing soap to smooth your enamel and gums... And the idea is gaining traction. The motive he prefers cleaning cleansing soap to toothpaste is that maximum toothpastes encompass glycerin, that would probably shape a coating at the enamel that calls for added than twenty rinses to put off. If the enamel is protected in a tough-to-get rid of coating, it will be no longer able to soak up the phosphate and calcium required for remineralization.

Dr. Judd claims that tooth cleansing cleaning soap receives rid of the coating from the tooth on the same time as moreover disinfecting the gums and killing any lingering micro organism. While premade tooth cleaning cleaning cleaning soap is available, it could be quite highly-priced. Making this possibility form of tooth cleanser at home is more inexperienced and price-powerful for maximum people. Here's a simple recipe in an effort to feed your complete family for at the least multiple weeks:

Ingredients for BASIC TOOTH SOAP:

•four teaspoons unscented liquid castile cleaning cleaning soap (together with Dr. Bronner's)

•half of cup bloodless-pressed virgin coconut oil, melted

•To taste, 1 to 2 teaspoons granulated birch xylitol or natural stevia extract

•25–30 drops antimicrobial crucial oil (peppermint, spearmint, cinnamon, or clove).

Fill the pitcher of your blender with 2 tablespoons of boiling water. Combine the soap, oil, sweetener, and essential oils in a blending bowl. Blend till the mixture is slight and frothy. In actually one among processes, transfer the tooth cleaning soap to a easy pump dispenser: Insert a funnel into the dispenser's top and press the cleansing cleaning cleaning soap in; instead, pour the soap proper proper into a huge plastic bag or icing bag, reduce open one small corner of the bag, and "pipe" the cleaning cleaning soap into the sphere.

To use enamel cleaning soap, squirt a small amount onto a moistened brush and exercise as you'll toothpaste.

If you do no longer have get right of access to to liquid castile soap or favor to use castile bar cleaning soap, make certain you do now not use hand-crafted cleaning soap due to the fact the glycerin in domestic made cleaning soap is commonly now not removed.

While it can take some time to get used to the taste and texture of tooth cleaning soap, you may be added directly to preserve the use of it once you see how whiter and extra wholesome your teeth are. One girl suggested that her family had normal bi-annual dental checkups and that now not one of the mother and father or their youngsters had a unmarried hollow space in the years at the same time as you recollect that the use of the tooth cleaning soap, eating a dental diet regime wealthy in raw milk, and supplementing with correct nutrients.

Previously, the mother pronounced that she may additionally get as a minimum one new hollow space each three hundred and sixty 5 days.

Chapter 14: Herbal Supplements For Healthy Teeth.

Cleaning enamel with tiny plastic bristles related to a plastic cope with is a extraordinarily new workout. People everywhere in the global had been cleaning their teeth with "chewing sticks" for masses of years.

The idea in the lower back of chewing sticks is that not amazing will chewing a fibrous twig scrape plaque off of tooth, but the stick itself is crafted from a plant with antimicrobial and antibacterial residences on the manner to kill germs before they infect the enamel.

CHEWING STICKS: The ends of twigs from small, fibrous timber are shredded and used to clean tooth surface and "floss" among enamel in plenty of tribal and rural cultures round the arena, specifically in Africa and South America. While many outstanding types of timber and timber have historically been used as chewing sticks, only a few have been scientifically studied for his or her dental efficacy.

Rhus vulgaris and lantana trifolia are two commonplace flora nonetheless utilized in developing countries for extensive tooth care, and every are being studied as a likely preference for presenting higher fitness care to the impoverished, as they will be a notable deal much less high priced and extra without trouble to be had than the plastic toothbrushes carried out in greater evolved industrialized elements of the place.

Rhus vulgaris is perception via using some of nicknames, which incorporates Quommo and Ongafire. This small shrub produces appropriate for ingesting berries and can be located sooner or later of Africa, from Cameroon to Ethiopia and south to Mozambique, Malawi, Zambia, and Zimbabwe.

Lantana trifolia, additionally known as "shrub verbena," is a broadleaf evergreen nearby to the West Indies, Mexico, Central and South America.

According to the authors of a cutting-edge have a examine posted in Front Pharmacol in 2011, customers of chewing sticks derived from those flora declare that:

•Cleaning posterior tooth with the stick is a whole lot much less tough than with a modern toothbrush because of the truth the pinnacle is smaller, and the tool is less complex to govern.

•The ease with which man or woman teeth can be cleaned reduces the prevalence of bleeding gums.

The sticks are pretty useful for scraping off plaque and particles. Researchers concluded that chewing sticks are a incredible opportunity to fashionable toothbrushes because of their innate antimicrobial houses.

With a renewed interest in opportunity dental fitness, dental chewing sticks are broadly to be had on the Internet and in some health food stores.

DENTAL HERBS: The herbalist network generally consents that food regimen is the most vital issue in teeth decay and, therefore, tooth health. As a give up give up result, the number one issue your herbalist will speak with you if you come to them for help together with your enamel is food. They can even ask you a chain of exceptional questions about everything out of your temper to your environment that lets in you to higher understand your specific makeup and scenario. An herbalist also can direct you to several specific herbs that would assist offer your body a teeth-constructing enhance after you have got were given been very well "examined" and your food regimen has been adjusted to growth the opportunity of remineralization and recuperation.

According to Christopher Hobbs, LAc, AHG, a herbalist and botanist with over thirty years of experience in herbal treatments, the subsequent herbs can useful aid inside the device of pathology reversal and tooth strengthening:

Resins with antibacterial and anti inflammatory houses

In addition to the precise houses listed under, the following resins have antibacterial and anti-inflammatory houses.

•Warming, astringent myrrh

•Propolis (bee product) stimulates the formation of new tissue and is antiviral.

•Propolis is mainly useful for mouth ulcers and sores.

•Pine resin (pitch)—When commercial enterprise corporation, it may be chewed like gum.

Herbs with Antimicrobial Properties

Usnea is a not unusual lichen that is greater powerful than penicillin toward streptococcus and staph.

Bloodroot is a plant neighborhood to the japanese woodlands that inhibits plaque and rot-inflicting micro organism.

Plantain, a not unusual "weed," may be used glowing to deal with abscesses.

Astringents (anti-microbial, tightens tissues)

These will assist to enhance your gums and solid the teeth.

Krameria has a tannin content material fabric of 40%. (antiviral). As a dentifrice for bleeding or spongy gums, integrate the powder with myrrh.

Tannins may be decided in as a great deal as 50% of very wellgalls (alrightapples). As a dentifrice, use powder.

Tormentil and Sage—Gargle for chronic gum infection.

Immune Stimulants

A robust immune tool guarantees that your frame produces and distributes nutrients to the teeth and gums for correct recovery and remineralization.

Baptisia—Antiseptic and anti-bacterial. Gargle or rinse with diluted tincture to set off community immunity and spark off recovery.

Aromatherapy Oils

Most essential oil-bearing vegetation can growth blood float to the gums, which permits power nutrients into the teeth. The following oils also are antibacterial, making them beneficial for disposing of ground micro organism:

Peppermint oil, Spearmint oil, Fennel oil, Cinnamon oil, Sage oil, Thyme oil, and Oregano oil are all crucial oils.

All those oils are without problems to be had at health food stores, can be ordered on-line, or may be received from your herbalist. To get the first-class outcomes, make certain your oil is of the awesome exquisite and purity.

Chapter 15: Orthodontics: How To Avoid Braces.

Braces appear like a ceremony of passage within the United States, particularly the diverse center and top schooling. When teens and children revel in enamel transferring, their dentist refers them for orthodontic remedy. Within a few years, their enamel is probably right away (without or with extractions, head tools, and different domestic equipment), their braces may be eliminated, and they'll be on their way—in all likelihood with some tooth decalcification.

Traditional braces straighten teeth by using applying low tiers of strain that are step by step manipulated to shift the teeth into the preferred alignment. Metal brackets are bonded right away to the teeth after which harassed out together and moved the use of elastics and is derived to accomplish this. Doesn't that sound like a cyborgsmile?

Braces usually charge among $3000 and $7000 and aren't normally blanketed via using dental coverage.

PLUS, there are a few side outcomes of braces that your dentist nearly in no way mentions, together with the fact that pushing the enamel causes enamel, bone, and root damage, that would motive gum ailment and root canals later in life. The capability risks of braces are usually cited in the wonderful print of your orthodontic settlement—however do you observe it?

Some dad and mom are searching out a more holistic and herbal way to straighten their tooth because of the excessive charge, extended device, look, or ache of conventional braces.

This is a extraordinary detail, due to the fact honestly placing braces on enamel does no longer deal with the underlying trouble: why are the tooth crooked inside the first place?

The solution lies in contemporary society's way of life. There are almost no examples of crooked tooth in primitive cultures or our pre-commercial organisation, pre-agricultural ancestors. This is thinking about their facial and jaw systems had been perfectly large enough to residence all of their enamel—no crowding! Dr. Weston Price positioned in his studies that the food regimen of these primitive humans became the number one thing in the lovely composition of their facial competencies and their wholesome, without delay enamel.

Now, ninety five% of people in countries in which processed modern factors dominate the diet plan have crooked teeth or misaligned jaws. It is critical to recognize that the connection amongst weight-reduction plan, jaw placement, and not unusual fitness is simple. According to Dr. Price's findings, natives with remarkably decay-unfastened tooth additionally had nicely-customary dental arches, ensuing within the wider, rounder face that is often related to fitness and beauty.

When a dental arch is properly aligned, the top and backside teeth are flush with every different—there may be no overbite or underbite. There will first-class be a hairline difference, with the top sticking out ever so barely to keep away from setting an excessive amount of pressure at the mandible.

The commonplace belief is that crooked and misaligned teeth are inherited.

Then we are able to throw up our arms and abdicate obligation. It's the easy (if not reasonably-priced) way out.

Our current jaws are disfigured because of a terrible diet lacking in important constructing blocks which consist of calcium and phosphorus. This is most apparent in the story of the Australian Aborigines. For heaps of years, era after generation, those tribal Aborigines reproduced with none sign of facial irregularities together with crooked, crowded teeth or misaligned jaws... Until the introduction of "white man's meals"—wheat flour, grain, and sugar—into their weight loss program. Suddenly, the youngsters evolved the equal dental arches and facial irregularities as youngsters from white civilizations.

The hyperlink amongst food plan and dental health exists and can't be left out any similarly.

So, how are we able to avoid having crooked teeth inside the first region? If you have look at this a protracted manner, you are likely aware of the solution: weight loss plan.

The key's to begin a nicely nourishing diet regime previous to concept, which means you and your partner eat this way as nicely. The earlier you begin nicely nourishing a growing fetus or child, the better the kid's opportunities of getting a well original jaw and sturdy, at once enamel.

Breastfeeding is recommended after the kid is born to maintain right jaw form and to provide good enough vitamins to growing bones and developing enamel.

This is an mainly essential time for the mom to nourish her personal body with the identical nutrient-wealthy, sugar-free food regimen. The fat-soluble vitamins and minerals will then be surpassed right now to the toddler thru breast milk, even as the mother will gain from a greater fit body and more potent tooth.

ARE YOUR TEETH ALREADY CROOKED? WHAT YOU SHOULD DO NOW:

Don't be alarmed if your very very personal or your infant's teeth are already crooked, or in case you take a look at an overbite or underbite. There are steps you could take to straighten your tooth and align your jaw whilst now not having to put on braces.

If your little one remains very younger, step one is to strictly adhere to the diet regime mentioned on this ebook. You can extensively alternate the development of the kid's chunk thru the food you provide him to nourish his body via way of using beginning the weight loss program as a toddler, as an entire lot as a 5- or six-12 months-vintage. If you're addressing specific issues, you can use homeopathic mineral salts each day.

Consult your homeopath about kinds and dosages, as anybody's chemical make-up varies, as do special factors along side age and weight.

Make high satisfactory your growing little one's weight loss program includes loads of uncooked milk products from grass-fed cows. Each u . S . Has its personal set of prison tips that govern the sale of uncooked milk. However, a smooth net look for "raw milk dairy" on your place will yield nearby farms an super manner to both allow for dairy-cow boarding or co-op milk. Ask around, investigate the farm, and get to recognize the farmer so that you may be assured the cows are being raised properly on a inexperienced pastured eating regimen and the milk is sanitary.

If you can not get raw milk products from the farm, raw cheeses are broadly to be had at fitness food shops and immoderate-forestall grocery stores.

In times of excessive jaw displacement or severely crooked teeth, older kids and adults want to are trying to find recommendation from a Dental Orthopedic. Unlike orthodontists, who're looking for to straighten teeth in any manner feasible, dental orthopedics are seeking out to realign the jaw and skull to their natural positions, allowing teeth to straighten in reality without using braces.

Instead of setting apart the enamel and jaw from the rest of the body, dental orthopedics considers the complete cranial shape. Furthermore, dental orthopedic medical scientific doctors apprehend the connection some of the cranial shape, jaw, and all of the body's complicated structures, all of that have an impact on every element of our health and properly-being. As you're conscious, we're holistic organisms that need to be regarded.

"All mechanical tensions positioned at the enamel might be contemplated into the cranial device and, if used by design, can serve to correct cranial lesions and enhance the affected person's incredible of lifestyles," says Dr. Gerald H. Smith.

What he says is extremely profound. Minor twine or appliance manipulations can practice pressure in locations on the way to then regulate exclusive physical systems, affecting everything from body shape to psychology.

All of this can be considered via your orthopedic dentist as he implements your remedy plan. Do you accept as real with that traditional orthodontists go through in thoughts what other systems (concerned? Cardiovascular? Digestive?) they'll have an effect on when they alter that cord or circulate that rubber band?

The chances are slender... Not because of the reality they do not CARE, however due to the fact it truly isn't how they've been taught.

A actual orthopedic practitioner might be able to have a observe your entire frame as an entire and contain bodywork which includes chiropractic and rubdown into your remedy plan.

Finding a person who appears past his or her personal area of information, however, may be tough. It may additionally ultimately be up to you to searching out out and take a look at out greater remedies to deal with the underlying reasons and remedies in your jaw misalignment.

Chapter 16: Natural Tooth Care: You Can Do It.

The most crucial takeaway from this book is that you aren't a bystander as regards to your dental health. You do not need to sit inside the dentist's chair like a victim, being lectured about oral hygiene in advance than being drilled and stuffed.

Stop blaming nature. Stop shrugging your shoulders and shopping for needless dental art work. Stop questioning that fillings and crowns are the identical detail.

Braces are an unavoidable part of developing older.

You have been given your self into this mess, and now you need to get yourself out of it.

YOU CAN heal and straighten your enamel. Food is the most powerful weapon for your arsenal.

I apprehend that this is a lot of information to soak up, and it'll maximum probable necessitate a entire shift to your ingrained beliefs approximately dental health. It's splendid. For your comfort, proper right here are the primary guidelines mentioned right here:

1. Consume a nutrient-dense diet plan that consists of pastured meat (together with organ meat), chicken, and eggs, uncooked and fermented pastured dairy, bone broth, seafood, and cod liver oil.

2. Avoid sugar and grains to your weight loss plan. This isn't always an alternative.

three. When important, supplement with homeopathic cell salts and herbs.

four. Get rid of toxic toothpaste. Instead, check with chewing gum, teeth cleansing cleaning cleaning soap, or clay toothpaste.

five. Consult an orthopedic dentist about jaw misalignment.

Following the ones clean steps will will will assist you to heal your teeth from the interior out, likely saving you loads of dollars in dental and clinical charges over your lifetime. You'll notice superb changes in every your mouth and your body in advance than you're privy to it.

Even in case you're in spite of the truth that skeptical, there can be no harm in giving it a shot. Making the ones small modifications is lots an awful lot less high priced than figuring out to shop for dental art work, a whole lot much less painful, and has no component results.

Your teeth will become whiter, harder, and shinier due to this remedy. Tooth pain will disappear, and the food regimen may additionally even benefit the rest of your body. You may also phrase which you are smiling greater and feeling better.

Chapter 17: What Is Teeth Decay And What Can It Do?

What is tooth decay?

Tooth decay is an infectious disease. The teeth enamel is the number one hit. A hollow space is fashioned in the tooth and then propagates in the direction of caries. If decay isn't dealt with, the hole receives large and decay can benefit the dentin (layer beneath the enamel). Pain starts offevolved offevolved offevolved to be felt, in particular with the recent, cold or sweet. The decay can win the pulp of the enamel. This is referred to as toothache. Finally, a enamel abscess might also moreover furthermore get up whilst the micro organism assault the ligament, bone or gum.

Sugars are one of the most essential chargeable for the assault on the teeth. Indeed, micro organism present inside the mouth, in particular the bacterium Streptococcus mutans and lactobacilli, sugars decompose into acids. They bind to acids, food debris and saliva shape so-known as dental plaque, the inspiration of dental caries. Tooth brushing gets rid of the plate.

Dental caries, very not unusual, affecting tooth (teeth decayed milk ought to be handled even though it is permitted to fall) and everlasting enamel. Rather they reap molars and premolars, which are extra difficult to clean at the same time as brushing. Cavities by no means heal spontaneously and may purpose teeth loss.

Diagnosis

The analysis is effortlessly made by means of the usage of the dentist due to the fact the decay is often invisible to the naked eye. He asks questions about ache and tooth sensitivity. An x-ray can verify the presence of a hole area.

Prevalence

Cavities are very commonplace. More than nine out of ten people would have had at least one hole area.

Caries affecting the crown of the teeth (the seen element that isn't blanketed by using the gums) will boom till midlife and then stabilizes. Caries affecting the premise of the enamel, frequently with the aid of way of the use of loosening or erosion of the gums, maintains to growth with age and are common inside the elderly.

Causes

The motives of teeth decay are multiple however the sugars, especially on the equal time as eaten among food are the number one culprits. For example, there is a hyperlink amongst sugary drinks and cavities or between honey and caries2. But wonderful factors on the side of snacking or wrong brushing of enamel also are implicated.

Complications

The decay may also moreover have vital consequences on the enamel and normal fitness. It can, as an instance, purpose intense pain, abscesses once in a while found through manner of manner of fever or swelling of the face, chewing issues and vitamins, tooth that wreck or fall, infections ... Caries must be cautious at the earliest.

Why you need to save you caries?

Symptoms

Symptoms of teeth decay are notably variable and depend specifically on the evolution of degradation and location diploma. At first, while the enamel is satisfactory reached, the decay may be painless. The most common symptoms are:

Toothache, which increase with time;

Sensitive teeth;

Severe pain while eating or ingesting some element bloodless, warm, sweet;

Pain while biting;

Brown spot at the enamel;

Pus across the teeth;

People at risk

Heredity performs a function in the improvement of caries. Children, children and the aged ought to expand extra frequently caries.

Risk Factors

The oral hygiene is a completely critical parameter in the improvement of dental caries. A diet plan immoderate in sugar furthermore drastically will growth the threat of developing cavities.

A loss of fluorine ought to moreover be accountable for caries. Finally, consuming troubles like anorexia and bulimia or gastro-esophageal reflux are conditions that weaken the enamel and make the installation of cavities much less complicated.

How to save you enamel decay?

The golden recommendations of dental hygiene

Cavities and gum illness answerable for tooth loss and painful and high-priced care can be prevented via pretty smooth every day hygiene. Do no longer hesitate to invite your dentist.

Although we are now more respectful of our dental hygiene, a few improvement remains feasible. What are the necessities to specific oral fitness policies?

Teeth, you Brush after each meal

Plaques, white sediment wherein micro organism proliferate, are causing caries and infection of the gums. As she is getting higher in some hours, it's far critical to eliminate it with the useful resource of brushing as a minimum instances each day.

A toothbrush with gentle bristles, nylon, you may pick and change them each 3 months

Brush scathing should injure the gums and harm the teeth of the enamel. A worn brush enamel is now not powerful. The electric powered powered toothbrushes can advantageously be used, furnished with often exchange of the surrender.

The proper method

Place the toothbrush 45 ° willing straddling the enamel and gums and brush alongside the teeth and gums, higher and reduce jaw one at a time, from the gum to the tooth with a rotary movement for three minutes.

Dental hygiene Use of dental floss, similarly to brushing removes dental plaque at the aspect faces of the tooth. For people who have free enamel or dentures that depart inaccessible brush areas, it's miles critical to use sticks or interdentally brushes; to take away dental plaque at the lowest of the enamel and stimulate the gum. The jet devices also are useful in this situation to remove meals particles, and massaging the gums.

The dentist

An annual visit to the dentist can discover early caries in time and could be an possibility to exercise scaling to do away with plaque. Two classes of scaling are reimbursed through social protection. But every so often extra is wanted. If plaque isn't detected in time, it grows intensive and paperwork a pocket a number of the bottom of the enamel and the gum, which might also quit result ultimately, loosening of tooth. At this degree, curettage underneath community anesthesia is wanted. It is not reimbursed with the useful resource of the usage of social security .

Attention to children

The enamel of our children are fragile and precious. To maintain enamel decay and one of a kind problems, right right here are a few suggestions to make certain them a colorful smile.

Dental grooves of your children, ye shall seal

In early life the risk of dental caries is mainly excessive. Eighty% in case the ones cavities growth in the grooves of the molars. By casting a fluid synthetic resin movie at the grooves, it is possible to prevent the ones cavities. This treatment can be completed at the output of the number one molars. It is covered through the usage of Social Security until age 14.

Chapter 18: A Dental Fitness Of Your Youngsters, You May Watch

The sugar water bottles or milk left at the small little one in bed at night time time time take their toll, leaving growing dental plaques and early caries. Similarly goodies need to be avoided at night time. Whenever viable, we have to choose candy or chewing sugarless gum.

Additional contributions of fluorine in the mom inside the path of being pregnant and childhood can be cautioned with the useful aid of the health practitioner to strengthen enamel. Finally, it is critical to tell the kid's use of the toothbrush, as more youthful as or 3 years.

To preserve wholesome teeth healthful, you want to have impeccable oral hygiene is a selection of toothpastes with very unique houses.

Anti-plaque and anti-bacterial

The problem: plaque is a deposit of meals debris and micro organism on tooth can be consistent. The sugars are converted into acids and could assault the enamel, growing cavities. Tissues are irritated gums inflicting gingivitis and untimely tooth loss.

The solution: Preferably use toothpaste that includes - a fairly excessive hobby - chlorhexidine, a effective anti-bacterial. He cleanses the mouth, facilitates combat bacteria and decreases the arrival of gingivitis. The movement is sluggish and lasts several hours.

Strengthens the teeth

The hassle: over the years, the tooth wears away, crumbles, is dematerialized because of the fact saliva is turning into scarcer. It end up she who irrigates enamel and offers calcium. The gums recede inflicting teeth loss and grade by grade lose their colour and shine.

The solution: a toothpaste containing calcium peroxide that rematerialize and strengthens teeth tooth whilst eliminating micro organism causing plaque. This molecule additionally has a bleaching impact and reduces floor stains. For extra overall performance, it's far beneficial to hold the toothpaste some time within the mouth in advance than rinsing.

Sensitive Teeth

The problem: this circumstance is manifested with the aid of ache quick however violent because of contact of the tooth to heat, bloodless, candy, acidic or maybe brushing. It is regularly due to a degradation of the neck of the enamel. The gums recede and denude the base of the teeth. The food contact is through the dentin to the nerve of the teeth, ensuing in ache.

The answer: A little abrasive gel or toothpaste that consist of little or fluorinol

Permethol that connect to the ground of the dentine and forms a protecting layer. Chlorhexidine additionally limits the bacterial proliferation is prolonged and after brushing. As a bonus those toothpastes can also shield your gums.

Brushing tooth is important to you!

You were pronouncing you're very small: you need to brush your tooth! But that has now not best correctly protected toward cavities. This each day gesture can preserve your lifestyles! Regular brushing protects your arteries and restriction the hazard of cardiovascular sickness.

Previously decided to be no longer dangerous, oral micro organism may be a good buy more insidious, causing inflammation of the arteries.

Bacteria which have a grudge toward your arteries

Brush brushing teeth cardiovascular disorder Several research had endorsed a hyperlink amongst the prevalence of cardiovascular illnesses and infections of the oral partitions 1 or lack of 2 teeth But a number of them a few of the most modern-day appeared to have questioned this speculation. While the scientific network is at the enamel, a big have a look at funded through way of the National five Institute of American Health (NIH) led by using Professor Desvarieux attempts to offer a definitive solution.

These researchers evaluated the big style of micro organism gift inside the mouth of 667 human beings, and at the same time, via Doppler ultrasound thickness of the carotid artery critical blood from the coronary heart to the top. This test is designed to hit upon atherosclerosis, a disorder characterised thru thickening and hardening of the arterial wall.

They positioned that people with the best presence of four unique bacteria, were folks that had the thicker arterial partitions. This relationship turn out to be impartial of different variables recognized to growth cardiovascular risk (age, diabetes, smoking, weight problems, and so on.).

We previously concept that those germs added about some gingivitis and other gum troubles. But further to issues of loosening, those stowaways need to consequently be lots greater sneaky. Especially due to the truth that the ones micro organism proliferate 6 in awful brushing.

Inflamed gums, swollen arteries!

How to hyperlink infection with those bacteria to atherosclerosis? The hyperlink most of the phenomena is contamination. The micro organism may additionally additionally furthermore input the bloodstream, and therefore excursion at some point of the frame. The immune tool then identifies as intruders and triggers neighborhood inflammations in the arteries, the walls swell and thicken.

This phenomenon of atherosclerosis have to he be able by myself to cause myocardial infarction or strokes? For now, it's miles a question that is hard to answer. But there are plans to re-have a have a observe the individuals in this have a have a look at to be aware the development of atherosclerosis.

Chapter 19: When Brushing Cleans The Arteries!

To save you the spread of those undesirable guests, the super solution is ideal dental hygiene. "Because periodontal infections may be without troubles prevented and treated, searching after his dental health ought to have a real impact on our cardiovascular health," said Professor. Desvarieux. In addition to taking your blood pressure, display screen your ldl ldl cholesterol, your blood sugar (diabetes), bodily interest and smoking conduct, your cardiologist need to fast show your dental hygiene.

Toothbrush for you

When did you purchase your toothbrush? If you do preserve in mind it's miles a horrible sign! What toothbrush chooses? Should we convert to electric powered powered toothbrush? The toothbrush you need.

The toothbrush in figures

Toothbrush 90 million toothbrushes are presented in America each 12 months. However, if the guidelines of the American Association for oral health had been found, this is to say, exchange the brush every 3 months, it's far 240 million toothbrushes that need to be used. We are an prolonged manner from...

To deal with his teeth, brushing has its significance. And who says unique brushing, stated exceptional toothbrush! So we can buy 4 toothbrushes constant with man or woman in keeping with yr, we "consume" 1.Five. Result: the brush wears out and is lots tons much less effective brushing. In quick, a toothbrush have to be modified regularly to keep it most flexibility, hygiene and software in opposition to plaque.

To every his toothbrush

If you often change the brush, it is also crucial to select cautiously. Each character has his little mouth troubles, and a toothbrush, it's miles very private. For kids, it need to be of a length and form tailor-made to their smaller than our personal mouth. And to decorate the exchange ought to now not hesitate to alternate colors and playful topics associated with those toothbrushes. For adults, it must understand the gums (hard enamel brushes are not endorsed), putting off plaque ... Adapt to the morphology to determine slip anywhere crucial.

Caries: prevention in location of undergo

It is the persistent disorder maximum common man. It impacts every enamel and everlasting enamel that men and youngsters as nicely.

Cavities are the primary enemy of our smile. Discover the four stages of the contamination that assaults our enamel and the manner to manage.

Stage 1: destruction of the teeth, no ache.

Stage 2: the dentine is attacked. Softer than enamel, it'll leave the sickness spread deeply. The heat, bloodless, candy and acid can cause pain.

Stage 3: bacterial invasion progresses and assault the pulp. Violent pains seem spontaneous is the toothache.

Stage four: The bacterial growth progresses to the tissues surrounding the tooth (ligament, bone, gum). It is the dental abscess. The cognizance of infection may be the purpose of the scenario remotely: microbes can migrate via the bloodstream inside the direction of the body, coronary coronary heart, sinuses, kidneys, eyes, joints ...

Tooth decay and meals

Previously, sugar have grow to be taken into consideration an remarkable and meals changed into reserved for patients or ate up at events. He have turn out to be a meals eaten every day for the improvement of business production of sugar, a century within the beyond. For a long term, enamel decay pleasant affected adults, and she or he or he began to reap out to children along with the improvement of the sugar enterprise.

Today it's miles a illness that in particular impacts youngsters, youngsters and teenagers; its frequency decreases after forty years. It is a public fitness problem that has a completely immoderate fee. In France, at the age of six years, -thirds of the kids already have as a minimum one hollow area.

Sugar and blend nicely caries

Tooth decay and caries healthy dietweight-reduction plan is a phenomenon of demineralization of hard tissues of the tooth (tooth, dentin, cementum), because of the acidic surroundings created thru the sugars furnished thru way of meals and a few micro organism in dental plaque. Sugar consumption is a key element within the formation of cavities. The maximum "cariogenic" sugars are sugars, together with sucrose, the number one element of sugar cane and beets. This is the maximum applied in confectionery. Followed with the useful resource of glucose (heavily produced corn, utilized in baking), fructose (fruit sugar), lactose (milk sugar) and starch (slow sugar grains and starches), which is a lot a remarkable deal less cariogenic.

An innate attraction to the candy taste

The taste for sugar is innate at start and the modern-day toddler select sugar water to herbal water. He prefers "strong" sugars, sucrose and fructose, sugars "vulnerable". This predominance for sweetness will grade by grade decrease with the purchase of latest flavors, sour is the longest relevant.

Long the sugar remains inside the toddler meals aside. It has a chilled impact and is the maximum stable manner to calm him down. Causing endorphins, it would lead to three dependence examined through manner of the hard weaning candy bedtime bottle ...

Hereditary cavities?

Sugar water and tremendous sugary liquids (sodas, juices) data to the little one bottle to feed him or soothe him at once answerable for the "little one bottle enamel decay." These a couple of cavities of the better teeth, because of prolonged contact of the sweet liquid at the enamel are normal of young kids.

Adolescents are observed "devastating decay" because of the fact young everlasting tooth are a lot less mineralized and allow the speedy development of caries, it surely is found out simplest at a very late degree.

The genetic inheritance of degradation is not proved; the frequency of caries in some families is as an alternative because of transmission of eating behaviors, with excessive consumption of candies in adolescents.

The sugar in children a immoderate symbolic and emotional rate: we praise or deprives kids candy ... It is tough to cast off sugar however may be restrained and particularly form the flavor other flavors.

Chapter 20: A Simple Herbal Remedy

To alkalize your entire mouth, study a few baking soda to your toothbrush. However, it isn't alternatively recommended to use every day or in massive quantities, however best after acidic meal, or while you experience contamination of your gums.

The vital oil of oregano

Oregano is a effective natural anti-bacterial, this is why we simplest use a drop of critical oil diluted in a tablespoon of vegetable oil for rinsing or brushing now and again. You can also dilute it with vegetable oil if you ever enjoy that he has too robust a taste.

plant

A herbal mouthwash

If you need to make your private mouthwash with natural way, so right here is an thrilling recipe this is especially primarily based totally on important oils:

materials:

3 drops of crucial oil of clove

10 drops of peppermint oil

3 drops tea tree vital oil

1 drop of crucial oil of cinnamon

3 drops of important oil of thyme

40 drops of liquor

a hundred ml of mineral water

Mix and stir all factors nicely, and preserve the mixture in a fab, dry place.

Avoid peppermint important oil if flushing is for kids.

Rinsing with seawater

For your mouthwash, there are bottles of purified sea water you could find in health food stores and herbalists. You ought to understand that sea water may be very alkaline and incorporates all of the essential minerals to your body.

People who live close to clean seashores also can convey straight away, however it is greater beneficial to do at dawn to keep away from when swimming, and try and fill the bottle to the lowest of the sea not taking the water returns to the floor, thereby to prevent residues which acquire there.

Hygiene is important: it's far what prevents the formation of plaque and bacterial movement.

Xylitol. Some studies5 suggested the effectiveness of xylitol in caries prevention. This herbal sweetener inhibit Streptococcus mutans. Chewing gums containing xylitol can be useful for tooth.

Propolis. Some animal exams have established promising outcomes in propolis, but in humans the effects are mitigés6. According to the author of a paper on anti-decay residences of propolis, the outcomes diverge because the composition of propolis used throughout varie7 trials.

Cheese. Cheese intake consistent with many studies need to prevent the onset of carie8,nine,10. Those accountable for this cariogenic effect can also need to cheese minerals, which include calcium and phosphorus. They save you tooth demineralization or even contribute to their minéralisation11. A study12 has advised his facet the effect on caries of yogurt consumption, but show the identical effects for unique dairy products like cheese, butter and milk.

Tea. Tea, whether or not or no longer black or inexperienced, would possibly moreover save you enamel decay. It ought to lower the movement of an enzyme found in saliva that role to degrade starch food into smooth sugars. Green tea have a beneficial effect on caries through its polyphenols that might restrict the increase of bacteria associated with carie13,14,15.

Cranberry. Cranberry consumption reduces plaque formation and dental caries. Prudence, but, because the juices comprise are frequently excessive in sugars and therefore terrible for the fitness buccale16.

Hops. Polyphenols, materials in hops, consistent with a few études17,18 gradual down the formation of plaque and consequently might make contributions to the prevention of caries.

Recap

Prevention is primarily based mostly on three interlocking factors:

Fluorine, given in addition to the early children to children with the resource of prescription dentist, improves resistance to teeth decay;

A strict oral hygiene and ordinary dental test-americaevery six months;

Limiting cariogenic sugars; that is the least well controllable component due to the reality sugar in all its forms is anywhere, in cabinets and fridges and in all locations that kids frequent. He continues a immoderate symbolic and cultural charge in a few populations. However, vitamins training gets results in caries prevention, mainly in better education. Like unique nutritional imbalance troubles (eg weight issues), decay have become a illness of poverty.

Chapter 21: Importance Of Dental Health

A easy and white smile plays a very important function in making someone's bodily appearance extra right. People who have a whole and healthy set of teeth normally normally tend to have higher arrogance than people who do now not.

They moreover tend to have more self guarantee and get jobs without troubles than folks that do not Poor dental fitness can also motive destiny economic burden due to expensive dental restoration strategies.

A whole set of tooth is likewise vital in speakme and ingesting. Your teeth are answerable for blocking off air from your mouth as you communicate. It is also important in cutting and grinding the meals you devour. It is essential inside the entire approach of digesting meals.

When you have got wholesome enamel, you can moreover make certain that you have wholesome gums. Healthy teeth also can contribute on how your breath might scent like.

Having healthy enamel additionally can help you avoid high exceptional diseases which includes diabetes, heart disease and infections.

Poor dental hygiene consequences in painful oral troubles that might affect the first-rate of your sleep and day by day sports activities. It moreover affects the right digestion of food.

It is essential that mother and father introduce right oral hygiene to their kids at the earliest possible age. Not best can this assist prevent cavities, but moreover keep away from the want to pay for steeply-priced dental prices within the future.

Proper oral hygiene includes the know-how of the right way of brushing tooth, flossing and rinsing the mouth. It additionally consists of the frequency of cleansing teeth and mouth every day.

Proper oral hygiene is vital due to the truth the lack of it may have an effect on the personal element, social detail and ordinary fitness of an character.

Poor oral fitness can also affect someone's right digestion. It can reason some digestive issues collectively with irritable bowel syndrome and intestinal issues.

Chapter 22: Guide To Basic Oral Hygiene

Proper oral hygiene is vital in someone's dental fitness. It is essential that someone is aware of proper oral hygiene physical activities. Through this, he can hold his teeth healthy, and avoid luxurious dental strategies.

Proper oral hygiene is tons less high priced in evaluation to dental strategies that need to be finished at the same time as you increase cavities.

The following are a number of the clean oral hygiene techniques that someone want to do to hold healthy mouth and enamel:

1. Visit the Dentist - It is important to have one or dental check-americayear as a manner to recognise the popularity of your oral health. If you feel a few factor one-of-a-kind to your teeth and gums, then you simply need to proper away time desk an appointment along with your dentist to have it checked.

2. Brush your Teeth Regularly - You must religiously comply with this number one step, brush and floss regularly. Though brushing and flossing 3 times a day is sufficient to preserve unique oral fitness, brushing and flossing after on every occasion you consume is a awesome deal higher. This way, you can make certain that you proper now dispose of the dust and micro organism out of your mouth and enamel.

Regular brushing and flossing can hold micro organism from multiplying and destroying your teeth. Using a mouth wash or rinse also can help flush out more dirt from the teeth and mouth.

3. Use a Soft-Bristled Toothbrush - Using a harsh toothbrush can scratch the ground of your tooth and make it weaker. To avoid this, use a easy-bristled toothbrush to make sure gentle cleansing.

four. Quit Smoking - Cigarette smoking is a hazard element in having enamel decay. Cigarette includes a few chemical substances that might be left on the tooth and live there honestly. These chemical materials could stick onto the tooth and spoil them.

Smoking furthermore contributes in growing terrible breath. If you can't give up smoking, then ensure to go to the dentist regularly for tooth cleansing or oral prophylaxis.

five. Eat Healthy - Eating nutritious substances can help make your enamel strong and save you teeth decay. Eating components rich in calcium could make stronger the enamel. Avoiding candy and sticky elements can assist save you tooth decay.

6. Replace your Toothbrush - To keep away from micro organism, you want to replace your toothbrush as fast as each three months. But in case you grow to be sick, you

want to replace it right away on the same time as you get over the infection. This manner, you could maintain your self from getting re-exposed to the bacteria that added about your contamination.

7. Air Dry your Toothbrush - When at domestic, permit your toothbrush to air dry, and do not keep it covered at the same time as wet. Covering it'll permit the micro organism to thrive in your toothbrush. If you prefer to have your toothbrush blanketed, then select one that have holes to allow air skip thru and dry it.

Letting your toothbrush dry in a toothbrush holder, or placing it in a cup upright can prevent micro organism formation.

Just cowl your toothbrush whilst you adventure to avoid it from rolling to your bag and selecting up germs from precise subjects.

Chapter 23: What Is Tooth Decay?

The loss of right oral hygiene can bring about dental troubles. One of the most common oral problems is teeth decay or the formation of cavities.

Cavities are damages at the tooth due to bacterial motion and the shortage of right oral hygiene. A cavity may be slight or really in the floor of the enamel. It additionally may be in a form of a pit. The maximum excessive form of hollow area is the nice that reaches the pulp and the muse of the tooth.

Cavities can motive pain to the affected man or woman. A immoderate case of hole region may be touchy at the same time as uncovered to cold or warmness liquids or food.

Tooth decay takes vicinity at the same time as the tooth lose minerals or whilst minerals aren't changed after an acid attack. The acid makes the ground of the teeth weaker and much less hard to erode.

After on every occasion you consume, an acid assault at the teeth follows straight away. The frame responds via the producing of saliva. The saliva includes minerals which encompass phosphate and calcium that update the minerals which have been washed out thru the acid. The saliva moreover counteracts with the acid and neutralizes it.

When someone does no longer have sufficient calcium in his weight-reduction plan, the remineralization of the tooth is probably affected. This might also moreover cause teeth decay.

When you eat, meals can stick onto the enamel and get caught into the spaces the various enamel and inner their corners.

If you do now not easy your enamel often, then those meals residues can shape a sticky movie or plaque on the enamel.

Plaque contains micro organism, that could convert carbohydrates into acid. The acid can wreck and erode the ground of the tooth.

It isn't unusual that small amounts of micro organism may be located in our mouth which includes lactobacillus and streptococci mutans. The immoderate amount of these micro organism in the mouth can increase the chance of teeth decay.

Frequent consuming of sugary substances (and not brushing and flossing) can motive the formation of cavities on the enamel. Sticky food which incorporates raisins or caramel can also boom the probabilities of the formation of cavities.

This additionally takes place whilst you eat acidic additives or drink acidic liquids which embody orange juice, grapefruit, beer, cola, pickles, vinegar and crimson wine.

Feeding a toddler to sleep can also motive cavities. The milk sits on the teeth for a long term, which lets in micro organism to supply acids which can reason enamel decay.

Plaque can smash enamel, similarly to the gums. This scenario is called gingivitis or infection of the gums.

People who smoke marijuana (hashish) or tobacco are extra vulnerable to have teeth decay. People who have intense alcoholism and weight issues are also at threat.

The shape and function of tooth can also increase the possibilities of enamel decay. If your enamel is shaped or located in a manner that it may with out difficulty trap meals residues, then you definitely actually want to pay near interest for your oral hygiene. You ought to ensure that you smooth your teeth thoroughly.

People with consuming problems together with anorexia and bullimia also are liable to enamel decay. In the mentioned situations, a person is much more likely to vomit often. The vomit consists of belly acids which could are available in contact with the tooth. Acid should make the enamel weaker and smooth to erode, consequently making them greater liable to hollow space formation.

People who snack in amongst meals (without brushing) are also extra at risk of cavities. The food residues can shape into plaque that incorporates bacteria. The micro organism can produce acids that can erode your enamel.

www.ingramcontent.com/pod-product-compliance
Lightning Source LLC
Chambersburg PA
CBHW060224030426
42335CB00014B/1332